OBJECTIVE STRUCTURED CLINICAL EXAMINATION IN OBSTETRICS & GYNAECOLOGY

This book is dedicated to Mrs Monica Bih Ntsambi
who died in 1978 from cervical cancer

Objective Structured Clinical Examination in Obstetrics & Gynaecology

JUSTIN C. KONJE
MD, MRCOG
Senior Lecturer in
Obstetrics & Gynaecology,
University of Leicester

DAVID J. TAYLOR
MD, FRCOG
Professor and Head of Department,
University of Leicester

**Blackwell
Science**

© 1998 by
Blackwell Science Ltd
Editorial Offices:
Osney Mead, Oxford OX2 0EL
25 John Street, London WC1N 2BL
23 Ainslie Place, Edinburgh EH3 6AJ
350 Main Street, Malden
    MA 02148 5018, USA
54 University Street, Carlton
    Victoria 3053, Australia
10, rue Casimir Delavigne
    75006 Paris, France

Other Editorial Offices:
Blackwell Wissenschafts-Verlag GmbH
Kurfürstendamm 57
10707 Berlin, Germany

Blackwell Science KK
MG Kodenmacho Building
7–10 Kodenmacho Nihombashi
Chuo-ku, Tokyo 104, Japan

The right of the Authors to be
identified as the Authors of this Work
has been asserted in accordance
with the Copyright, Designs and
Patents Act 1988.

First published 1998

Set by Semantic Graphics, Singapore
Printed and bound in Great Britain
by MPG Books Ltd, Bodmin, Cornwall

DISTRIBUTORS

    Marston Book Services Ltd
    PO Box 269
    Abingdon, Oxon OX14 4YN
    (*Orders*: Tel: 01235 465500
                    Fax: 01235 465555)

USA
    Blackwell Science, Inc.
    Commerce Place
    350 Main Street
    Malden, MA 02148 5018
    (*Orders*: Tel: 800 759 6102
                    781 388 8250
                    Fax: 781 388 8255)

Canada
    Login Brothers Book Company
    324 Saulteaux Crescent
    Winnipeg, Manitoba R3J 3T2
    (*Orders*: Tel: 204 224-4068)

Australia
    Blackwell Science Pty Ltd
    54 University Street
    Carlton, Victoria 3053
    (*Orders*: Tel: 3 9347 0300
                    Fax: 3 9347 5001)

A catalogue record for this title
is available from the British Library

ISBN 0-632-04764-X

The Blackwell Science logo is a
trade mark of Blackwell Science Ltd,
registered at the United Kingdom
Trade Marks Registry

For further information on
Blackwell Science, visit our website:
www.blackwell-science.com

CONTENTS

Part C: Neonatology

Part D: Revision Questions

Colour plates fall between pp. 86 and 87

CONTRIBUTORS

KARIN WILLIAMSON
FRCS, MRCOG
Consultant Gynaecologist
City Hospital Nottingham

SANDIE BOHIN
MRCP
Consultant Neonatologist
Leicester Royal Infirmary

PREFACE

There has been a recent trend towards testing clinical competence, the Objective Structured Clinical Examination (OSCE), since the original description by Harden and colleagues in 1986. This development is in recognition of the deficiencies in the long- and short-case clinical examinations. Not only have many medical schools introduced the OSCE to assess clinical competence but many postgraduate colleges around the world are gradually introducing them.

Many candidates will be encountering the OSCE type of examination for the first time. For others who might have sat the OSCE examination as medical students, there is a deficiency of information to assist with the preparation for this type of examination.

This book is aimed at the candidate preparing for OSCE examinations in Obstetrics and Gynaecology. It will be particularly useful for medical students and for candidates preparing for the Diploma in Obstetrics and Gynaecology of the Royal College of Obstetricians and Gynaecologists. Those candidates preparing for the MRCOG or equivalent examinations will hopefully find this book helpful during their preparations for the clinical and oral examinations. It is possible that this type of examination may be introduced into the MRCOG examination in the future. Teachers and examiners may also find this book useful, particularly the guidelines describing how to organize an OSCE examination and what type of questions to set.

We recognize that the standards of some of the questions will be higher than that expected of a medical student or a DRCOG candidate. In addition, there are some controversial questions and certainly some controversial answers. The opinions expressed are purely ours and we accept responsibility for the answers although others may disagree with them. It would not be Obstetrics and Gynaecology if there were no controversies!

ACKNOWLEDGEMENTS

We would like to thank Mr Roger Neuberg FRCOG (Consultant Obstetrician and Gynaecologist), Mr Joseph Emembolu FRCOG (Consultant Gynaecologist), Mr Victor Chilaka MRCOG (Urogynaecologist), Mr Sunday Ikhena MRCOG (Specialist Registrar), Dr Gill Wandless (Senior Medical Officer, Family Planning) and Dr Christine Cordle (Clinical Psychologist) for going through some of the questions and making useful comments and corrections.

We are grateful to Dr Laurence Brown (Consultant Histopathologist), Dr Vincent Riley (Consultant, Genitourinary Medicine) and Dr Patricia MacKever (Consultant, Paediatric Pathology) for some of the photographs/images used in this book.

INTRODUCTION

The two main objectives of medical examinations are to test (i) factual knowledge and (ii) clinical competence. The latter includes the ability to communicate effectively and empathically, counsel non-judgementally, elicit appropriate physical signs and perform practical procedures. The traditional methods of assessment – multiple choice, essay and short-answer questions – are able to test factual knowledge but there has been considerable concern about the ability of the long and short clinical case to assess clinical competence of candidates (Wilson *et al.* 1969). Some of the shortcomings of these traditional methods of testing clinical competence have included the lack of sensitivity, the broad spectrum of clinical cases used, the restricted scope for assessment, difficulties with the objective assessment of history taking, communicative and counselling skills and the wide variation in standards of the examiners and their perception of what is to be tested (McFaul *et al.* 1993).

In 1975, Harden *et al.* described an alternative form of assessing clinical competence. This type of examination was called the 'Objective Structured Clinical Examination' more commonly known by its acronym OSCE. This type of examination is designed to try and eliminate the shortcomings of the traditional examination methods and to try and improve the reliability and validity of the examination as a means of assessing clinical competence. In some examinations it has completely replaced the clinical examination while in others it complements it.

What constitutes an OSCE

The OSCE examination is aimed at testing various aspects of clinical competence. These include:
1 history taking;
2 physical examination to elicit clinical signs;
3 factual knowledge;
4 interpretation of laboratory results and clinical data;
5 recognition of pathology;
6 ability to formulate differential diagnoses;
7 counselling skills;
8 clinical problem solving;
9 effective prescribing of drugs and explanation of their side-effects;
10 use of instruments.

These aspects are assessed in a circuitry set-up with each station testing different aspects of clinical competence. The number of stations varies and most circuits include communication stations. At these interactive stations, the candidates may meet role-players who may present as patients with specific problems which may require diagnosis, or an examiner who may play the part of a patient or the part of another professional with identified roles, or a relative of a patient. At some stations the candidates are given a rest and these are commonly situated close to the interactive stations. The assessment at each interactive station or those where the candidates are expected to perform a specific task/procedure can be made on a form to standardized levels of competency.

1

The examination

The OSCE examination consists of several stations contained in one circuit. The number of stations in a circuit vary – the larger the number the greater the reliability of the examination. There are 22 stations at the Diploma in Obstetrics and Gynaecology examination (DRCOG).

At each station, a specific clinical competence is tested. The candidate is provided with written information in the form of a question, and there will be associated clinical data, photographs, charts, laboratory results, a person to interact with, etc. The information at the station is not expected to be removed from the station. If written answers are required, then either a standard answer sheet for each station or an answer booklet which the candidate carries around during the examination is provided.

There is no strict time-limit for a station, but each station should last about the same length of time otherwise the examination will be impossible to coordinate. Those setting the exam may decide, for example, to make each station last 4–10 minutes. A timekeeper will sound a bell at the end of each time period and the candidates should then move onto the next station where they answer the next question or perform the set task. For the DRCOG, the time spent at each station is six minutes.

When the candidates reach the interactive stations, they are provided with information upon which the discussion, counselling, history taking, etc., will be based. For effective assessment at this station, it is better for the candidates to have had this information at a rest station before the interactive station so that they can think clearly about it and formulate how to logically approach the task expected of them. If the station involves a role-player, there will usually be an examiner who observes and assesses the performance of the candidate. Occasionally the role-player may also be the assessor. This presents difficulties if the role-player is not a medical doctor or is a junior without enough ability to assess the candidate's performance.

Organization of an OSCE examination

The objective of an OSCE examination is to assess clinical competence across a broader range of competencies than is possible by the traditional long- and short-case clinical examination. Planning is therefore very important. Selby *et al.* (1995) identified seven important steps in the development of an OSCE examination. Of the seven steps, the six most important are the determination of:
1 the skills to be assessed;
2 the number of stations required to assess these skills
3 how these skills are to be assessed;
4 what marking scheme will be adopted;
5 what type of personnel will be required;
6 where the examination will take place.
When deciding on the number of stations, therefore, it is important to determine the minimum skills expected from an average candidate. The minimum number of stations within the circuit should cover all these minimum skills. Selby *et al.* (1995) recommended a miminum of 10 stations. At the DRCOG there are usually 22 stations. However, additional stations may be added to enable discrimination between poor, average and very good students.

The next important issue that needs to be addressed is how these skills are to be assessed. It is important that a uniform assessment format is adopted for each candidate. These may differ with the stations. For the DRCOG, the candidates are given an answer booklet containing a sheet for each station. Each question contains subsections and a limited number of boxes in which to write the answer. The boxes limit what a candidate can write. The answers are either correct or incorrect.

Because of the nature of medicine, many stem questions have more answers than the space provided could contain. This gives the candidate some room for manoeuvre. At the interactive stations, there are marking sheets for the examiners and the role-players.

For this type of examination to be objective, a standardized form of marking is required. A multiple choice format is one way of achieving this. If free text answers are required, then the candidates must be prevented from providing vague and lengthy answers. A way of doing this is by limiting the space for the answers. The DRCOG provides answer booklets with spaces in which the candidates must enter their answers. Where stems of questions require more than one answer, boxes can be provided for each of the stems equivalent to the number of answers required. Candidates must be instructed that they are not to write outside the boxes. This will ensure that the marking is fairly consistent. An example of this type of an answer sheet is shown right.

At the interactive station, the marking sheet should reflect the particular skill being assessed. If the station is assessing the candidate's communication skill, then emphasis must not be placed on factual knowledge. Having said that, it is important not to forget that this is a medical examination and therefore communication should be within the context of the discipline. Use of appropriate language, eye contact and the general mannerism of the candidate must be assessed. Since the rapport the candidate establishes with the patient role-player is very important, a question which enquires whether the patient role-player will be prepared to see the candidate again is often included. An example of a typical marking sheet for this type of station is shown on p. 4.

Sample question and answer sheet

Write your answer in the space provided. *Do not* write outside the space.

Question 1 A 26-year-old nulliparous woman has just had a diagnostic laparoscopy and extensive endometriosis has been diagnosed.

a. What four symptoms might she have presented with?

....
....
....
....

b. What three medical treatment options might you offer?

....
....
....

c. What three theories have been advanced for the occurrence of endometriosis?

....
....
....

d. What advice would you give her about fertility?

....
....

Sample interactive question and marking sheet

Question 2 A 27-year-old teacher was referred to a gynaecologist because of threatened miscarriage at seven weeks' gestation. An ultrasound scan showed an absent fetal heart beat and an irregular gestational sac. Could you advise her please.

Typical marking sheet

Aspect being assessed	Score = 0	Score = 0.5	Score = 1
Introduction			
Appropriate eye contact			
Explanation in a way that patient comprehends (avoiding technical language)			
Encouraging and answering questions			
Empathy/sympathy			
Outlining management options			
Would role-player like to see candidate again?			

These examples are not prescriptive. They
have to adapted depending on the station.

References

Harden R., Stevenson M., Downie W. W. & Wilson G. M. (1975) Assessment of Clinical
    Competence using Objective Structured Examination. *British Medical Journal*, i,
    447–451.
McFaul P. B., Taylor D. J. & Howie P. W. (1993) The Assessment of Clinical Competence
    in Obstetrics and Gynaecology in 2 Medical Schools by an Objective Structured Clinical
    Examination. *British Journal of Obstetrics and Gynaecology*, 100, 842–846.
Selby C., Osman L., Davis M. & Lee M. (1995) Set up and run an Objective Structured
    Clinical Exam *British Medical Journal*, 310, 1187–1189.
Wilson G. M., Lever R., Harden R. M. & Robertson J. D. (1969) Examination of Clinical
    Examiners. *Lancet*, i, 37–40.

Part A
Gynaecology

QUESTIONS

Menstrual disorders

1 A 26-year-old teacher presented with
scanty periods of 12 months' duration. Her
periods were regular and normal until she
had an evacuation for an incomplete
miscarriage.
a. What is the likely diagnosis?
b. What two investigations might you
    perform to confirm your diagnosis?
c. What treatment might you offer this
    patient?
d. What three complications may occur in
    pregnancy?

2 A 32-year-old woman has been told that
she is suffering from premenstrual
syndrome. She has come to see you for
counselling with some questions and a
diary which you requested her to keep.
a. How will you confirm that she is
    indeed suffering from premenstrual
    syndrome?
b. Which four physical symptoms may she
    be experiencing?
c. Which four treatment options might
    you offer her?
d. What is the risk of her developing
    postnatal depression if she becomes
    pregnant?
e. What is the risk of her children
    suffering from premenstrual syndrome?

3 Mrs JCK is 28 years old. She is suffering
from painless heavy but regular menstrual
cycles. A pelvic examination was
unremarkable and an ultrasound scan did
not reveal any abnormal pelvic organ.
a. What other three investigations would
    you like to perform on her?
b. What is the condition called?
c. Which four treatment options might
    you offer her?

d. If she has completed her family and
    medical treatment fails, what other two
    options might you offer her?

4 A 19-year-old girl has been referred to
you with failure to commence
menstruation. The mother tells you that
she had a prenatal diagnosis because of a
small swelling behind her daughter's neck
at 16 weeks and that she was told that her
chromosomes are 45XO.
a. What is the name for this condition?
b. Which five clinical signs might you
    elicit?
c. Which two important observations may
    be made at laparoscopy?
d. Which treatment will you offer her and
    why?
e. What advice will you offer her about
    her future fertility?

5 A 43-year-old woman presents with
irregular and heavy periods for six months.
She has had two children and was sterilized
six years ago. Her last cervical smear
performed six months ago was normal.
Apart from a bulky uterus, there was no
other abnormality. A full blood count
revealed a haemoglobin level of 11.5 g/dl.
a. What three important investigations
    will you perform on her?
b. The investigations fail to reveal any
    abnormality. What is the most likely
    diagnosis?
c. What is likely to be the medical option
    you offer her?
d. If the histology report revealed atypical
    endometrial hyperplasia, what treat-
    ment advice will you offer her and
    why?

6 Figure 1 (see also colour plate section,
facing p. 86) is a photograph from an

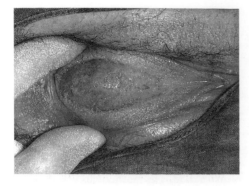

Fig. 1

18-year-old girl complaining of primary amenorrhoea. She has a normal female phenotype.
a.　What is the diagnosis?
b.　What other five symptoms may she present with ?
c.　What other investigation might you perform on her?
d.　What treatment will you offer her?
e.　What is her genotype likely to be?

7　A two-week-old neonate was diagnosed as having external ambiguous genitalia at birth as it was difficult to ascertain whether the gender was male or female. A similar problem was encountered with the older sib.
a.　What investigations will you perform on the neonate?
b.　What is the most important immediate step that must be taken to reduce morbidity?
c.　The karyotype is 46XX and examination under anaesthesia has not revealed any abnormality, but the 17-alpha-hydroxyprogesterone is raised. What is the diagnosis?
d.　What is the pattern of inheritance for this condition?
e.　What will be your two long-term management plans?

Early pregnancy disorders

1　Mrs TDB is 22 years old and presents with excessive vomiting for the past four days. Her last menstrual period was seven weeks ago and a urinary pregnancy test is positive.
a.　What is the most likely diagnosis?
b.　List four abnormal conditions that may be associated with this condition.
c.　Which four important investigations would you like to perform on her?
d.　What complications may result from this condition?

2　A young woman presented to the accident and emergency department with eight weeks of amenorrhoea, vaginal bleeding for three days and a temperature of 38.5°C. A pelvic examination revealed an offensive bloody vaginal discharge and an opened cervical os.
a.　What is the most likely diagnosis in this patient?
b.　What two other clinical signs might you elicit on examination?
c.　What five investigations will you perform on her?
d.　How will you manage the patient?
e.　What three complications may arise from this condition?
f.　Which three organisms may be isolated from this patient?

3　Mrs Smith is nine weeks' pregnant and presented with painless vaginal bleeding of two days' duration. The cervical os was closed and the uterus was enlarged to the size of an eight-week gestation at vaginal examination. The adnexa were non-tender.
a.　What are the two most likely diagnoses?
b.　What single investigation will you perform to distinguish between the two differentials? What will the difference be?

c. What other single investigation will you perform on the patient and why?

d. How will you manage these differentials?

4 An 18-year-old female presents with abdominal pain of three hours' duration, six weeks' amenorrhoea, a positive home pregnancy test and vaginal bleeding.

a. Which six physical signs might you elicit?

b. What four investigations might you perform?

c. What are the likely differential diagnoses?

d. What are the treatment options for two of your differential diagnoses?

5 Figure 2 (see also colour plate section) is a specimen taken at surgery from a 26-year-old single mother of two who presented with irregular dark brown vaginal bleeding, lower abdominal pain and a raised beta-human chorionic gonadotrophin (β-HCG).

a. What is the most likely diagnosis?

b. Give four predisposing factors to this condition.

c. Which are the two most common methods of confirming the diagnosis of this condition?

d. What advice will you give the patient before she leaves the hospital?

6 A young girl of 16 with three sexual partners has come to you requesting termination of pregnancy at seven weeks' gestation. She has been seen by a counsellor and is going ahead with the termination but has the following questions for you.

a. How will the procedure be performed?

b. What are the possible long-term effects of the termination on her future fertility?

c. What investigations will be performed before the procedure?

d. What other important advice will you give the girl?

7 Figure 3 (see also colour plate section) shows a specimen evacuated from the uterus of a young girl at 13 weeks' gestation.

a. What is the pathological condition?

b. What three symptoms may she have presented with?

c. What three signs may be elicited?

d. After treatment, what would the long-term management be?

e. What two reasons are necessary for long-term follow-up?

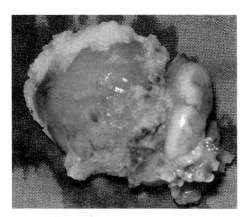

Fig. 2

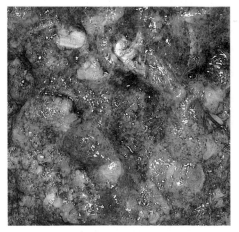

Fig. 3

8 The patient is a 22-year-old unmarried secretary. She has had one termination of pregnancy and is currently not on any form of contraception. Her last menstrual period was 10 days ago but she has been experiencing lower abdominal pain of increasing severity and associated irregular vaginal bleeding. Her abdomen is tender, with associated guarding and rebound tenderness. The cervix is closed but she is extremely tender in the right adnexum.
a. What are the three most likely differential diagnoses?
b. Which four investigations will you perform to distinguish between these differentials?
c. What treatment will you offer for each of your differentials?

9 A 26-year-old presented to the gynaecology unit with six weeks' amenorrhoea, abdominal pain and vaginal bleeding. A diagnosis of an incomplete miscarriage was made and she subsequently had an evacuation of the uterus under general anaesthesia. The histology report was as follows 'scanty fragments of endometrial tissues showing hypertrophy of the glands and oedema of the stroma. There is infiltration with polymorphonuclear leukocytes. No chorionic villi are seen'.
a. What is the phenomenon called?
b. In what two conditions may this be a feature?
c. What further plan of management will you offer this young woman?
d. If she continues to have pain, what important procedure might you perform?

10 Mrs Fisher has had three miscarriages. The first one was at six weeks, the second at 10 weeks and the third at 20 weeks' gestation. On all three occasions, the miscarriage was preceded by vaginal bleeding, abdominal pain and the passage of 'liver-like' tissues.

a. What is the diagnosis?
b. What is the most likely uterine cause of this condition?
c. What three investigations might you perform on her?
d. What treatment may she be offered?
e. What is the long-term prognosis?

Infertility and gynaecological endocrinology

1 A 26-year-old nulliparous woman is complaining of infertility. There is no relevant past medical history. Progesterone assays indicate that she is ovulating and her husband's semen analysis is normal. She has had an investigation shown in Fig. 4.
a. What is the investigation shown?
b. What has been revealed by this investigation?
c. Which are the two most common microorganisms responsible for this condition?
d. Give three other likely causes for this.

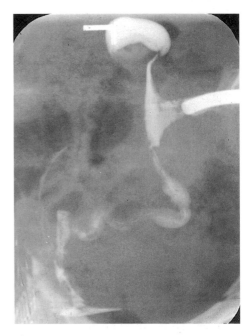

Fig. 4

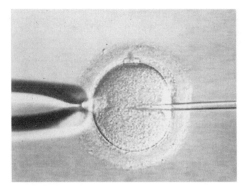

Fig. 5

e. Which treatment option is most likely to be successful in resolving her infertility?
f. Which non-treatment option may the couple consider?

2 Figure 5 shows a type of infertility treatment.
a. What is this type of infertility treatment called?
b. Give two indications for this form of treatment.
c. If the couple did not wish to progress to such complex treatment, which two alternatives may be available to them?
d. What is the success rate of the treatment shown in Fig. 5 where the husband is azoospermic?

3 GIFT is a form of infertility treatment.
a. What does the acronym GIFT stand for?
b. For GIFT to be carried out instead of *in vitro* fertilization and embryo transfer (IVF-ET), what absolute prerequisite must be satisfied?
c. Before eggs and sperms can be used for assisted reproduction treatments, what absolute requirement must first be fulfilled under the terms of the Human Fertilisation and Embryology Act 1990?

d. A couple can elect to store (by cryopreservation) embryos from an IVF-ET programme which are surplus to their immediate transfer requirements. Give two ways in which the couple may have initially decided the embryos should be used in the future should one of them die or become mentally incapacitated.

4 A 32-year-old woman has been having irregular menstrual cycles for six years and has been also trying to conceive for four years. Her husband's semen analysis is normal. Her thyroid function test and tubal patency test are normal.
a. What is the most likely diagnosis?
b. What additional three clinical signs might be present?
c. What two important investigations might you perform on her?
d. What is the likely cause of her infertility?
e. By what methods might you treat her infertility?

5 A 22-year-old single medical student presented with irregular periods of two years' duration. She is not obese. A blood hormone profile was performed and the results shown in the report (Fig. 6) were obtained.
a. What is the likely cause of the irregular periods?
b. What other symptoms may she present with?
c. List three methods by which you may treat the hirsutism.
d. What are the possible long-term medical complications of this condition?
e. In the absence of hirsutism, what is the best means of regulating her periods?
f. What future advice will you give her?

6 Mrs FT has secondary amenorrhoea. She has been investigated and her

W360	LEICESTERSHIRE PATHOLOGY SERVICE			
	CHEMICAL PATHOLOGY			

Cons/GP & Location:	UNIT NUMBER:		SURNAME:
	DoB/Age: 22 years	Sex: F	Forename:
	Patient Address:		

Specimen type:	Lab No:	Date & Time of report:

```
        FSH              = 3.7 iu/l
        LH               = 18.4 iu/l
        Prolactin        = 250 mu/l
        Estradiol        = 870 pmol/l
        Progesterone     = 7.5 nmol/l
        Androstenedione  = 18.4 nmol/l
        Testosterone     = 1.6 nmol/l
```

Comment:

Diagnosis:

T Bilirubin μmol/l 3-17	Alan. Trans. IU/l 2-53	Gamma G.T. IU/l 0-35f;50m	Alk. Phos. IU/l 40-130	Urate μmol/l 200,350f;500m	Phosphate mmol/l 0.8-1.4	T. protein g/l 60-80	Albumin g/l 35-55	Adj. Calcium mmol/l 2.1-2.6
Sodium mmol/l 133-144	Potassium mmol/l 3.3-5.3	Bicarbonate mmol/l 22-30	Urea mmol/l 2.5-6.5	Creatinine μmol/l 60-120	Calcium mmol/l 2.1-2.6	Glucose mmol/l 4.0-6.6	Date & Time of Specimen	

QUOTED REFERENCE RANGES ARE FOR ADULTS

Fig. 6

endocrine profile is shown in the laboratory report (Fig. 7).
a. What is secondary amenorrhoea?
b. What is the likely cause of her problem?
c. What other investigation would you like to perform on her?
d. Assuming this investigation is negative, which drugs might you offer her?
e. How will you prescribe these drugs?
f. Give four other causes of this type of amenorrhoea.

7 This report (Fig. 8) is from a 35-year-old husband of a 20-year-old woman who has been complaining of infertility for 18 months.
a. What do the results show?
b. What would be your next line of management?

c. What further steps would you take after (b)?
d. What three options of treatment may the couple benefit from?
e. If there were no sperms on this report, what two investigations will you need to perform?

8 Mr and Mrs Smith have been to an IVF clinic for evaluation for assisted conception. Mrs Smith is ovulating regularly as evidenced by normal menstrual cycles and luteal phase progesterone levels. Her tubes have also been shown to be patent on HyCoSY. Mr Smith's semen analysis is shown in Fig. 9.
a. What is wrong with Mr smith's semen analysis?
b. What five conditions may be responsible for this result?

LEICESTERSHIRE PATHOLOGY SERVICE
CHEMICAL PATHOLOGY

W360

Cons/GP & Location:	UNIT NUMBER:
	DoB/Age: 32 years Sex: F Forename:
	SURNAME:
	Patient Address:

Specimen type:	Lab No:	Date & Time of report:

```
FSH              = 6.5 iu/l
LH               = 7.4 iu/l
Prolactin        = 1 500 mu/l
Androstenedione  = 6.4 nmol/l
Oestradiol       = 570 pmol/l
Progesterone     = 18 nmol/l
```

Comment:

Diagnosis:

T Bilirubin μmol/l 3-17	Alan. Trans. IU/l 2-53	Gamma G.T. IU/l 0-35f;50m	Alk. Phos. IU/l 40-130	Urate μmol/l 200,350f;500m	Phosphate mmol/l 0.8-1.4	T. protein g/l 60-80	Albumin g/l 35-55	Adj. Calcium mmol/l 2.1-2.6

Sodium mmol/l 133-144	Potassium mmol/l 3.3-5.3	Bicarbonate mmol/l 22-30	Urea mmol/l 2.5-6.5	Creatinine μmol/l 60-120	Calcium mmol/l 2.1-2.6	Glucose mmol/l 4.0-6.6	Date & Time of Specimen

QUOTED REFERENCE RANGES ARE FOR ADULTS

Fig. 7

c. Which two investigations will you perform to distinguish between these causes?

d. What treatment options may be available for this couple?

9 The temperature chart shown in Fig. 10 was obtained from a 28-year-old nulliparous woman who has been attending her GP for 18 months for infertility.

a. What is the likely diagnosis from the chart?

b. What further three investigations might you perform to confirm the diagnosis?

c. What three conditions may cause this problem?

d. Where there is no identifiable cause, how may it be corrected at first?

e. What are the two complications of this initial correction?

10 A 30-year-old woman presented with infertility of three years' duration. Her menstrual cycle has been regular. Abdominal and pelvic examinations were all normal. A temperature chart for the past three months and her husband's semen analysis from her GP were normal.

a. What single additional investigation would you like to perform?

b. By which three methods may this test be performed?

c. What are the advantages and disadvantages of these methods of investigation?

d. Which additional baseline investigations might you perform?

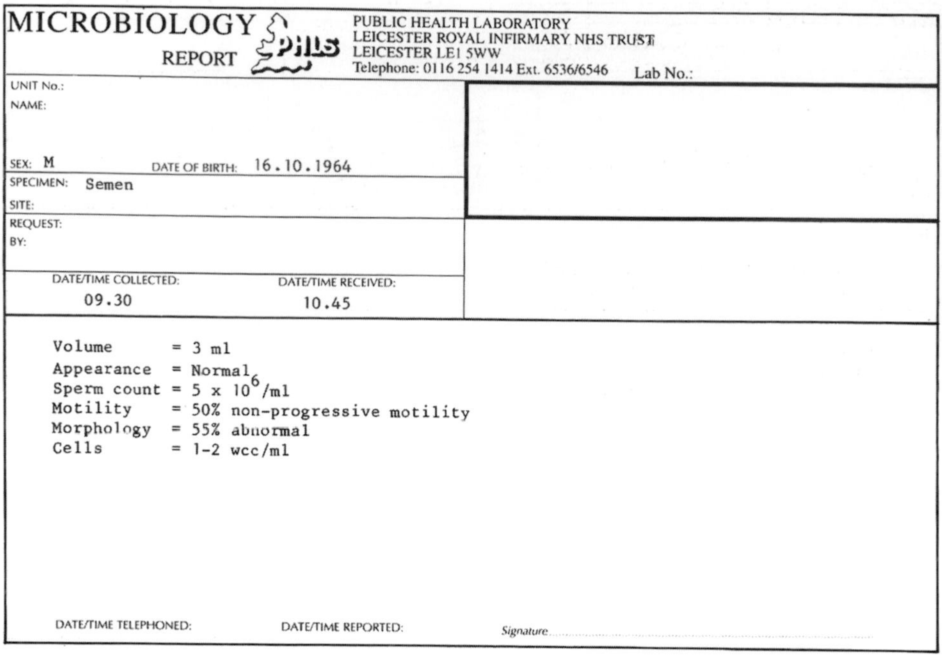

```
MICROBIOLOGY                    PUBLIC HEALTH LABORATORY
                                LEICESTER ROYAL INFIRMARY NHS TRUST
              REPORT            LEICESTER LE1 5WW
                                Telephone: 0116 254 1414 Ext. 6536/6546    Lab No.:
UNIT No.:
NAME:


SEX: M              DATE OF BIRTH:  16.10.1964
SPECIMEN:   Semen
SITE:
REQUEST:
BY:

    DATE/TIME COLLECTED:         DATE/TIME RECEIVED:
         09.30                        10.45


    Volume      = 3 ml
    Appearance  = Normal
    Sperm count = 5 x 10⁶/ml
    Motility    = 50% non-progressive motility
    Morphology  = 55% abnormal
    Cells       = 1-2 wcc/ml




    DATE/TIME TELEPHONED:        DATE/TIME REPORTED:      Signature
```

Fig. 8

Endometriosis

1 This photograph (Fig. 11, see also colour plate section) was taken at a laparoscopy performed on a 30-year-old nulliparous woman.
a. What is the likely diagnosis?
b. What three symptoms may she have presented with?
c. What associated condition may she present with?
d. What four treatment options might you offer this patient?
e. Give three theories about the origin of this condition.

2 A 27-year-old woman has been referred because of painful periods.
a. What relevant questions will you ask to help you make the correct diagnosis?

b. What clinical signs might you elicit to help in your differentials?
c. What single investigation will you perform to confirm your diagnosis?
d. What are your three differential diagnoses?

3 Mrs Brown has been suffering from lower abdominal pain and severe deep dyspareunia for six years. The findings at diagnostic laparoscopy performed six weeks ago demonstrated endometriosis on the uterosacral ligaments and ovaries. She went home on danazol and has come to see you for follow-up with a few questions.
a. How common is this condition?
b. Can this condition affect her future fertility?
c. What other three medical treatment alternatives may she be offered?
d. What four temporary side-effects of danazol may she have?
e. What if she is planning to become pregnant?

```
MICROBIOLOGY          PUBLIC HEALTH LABORATORY
                      LEICESTER ROYAL INFIRMARY NHS TRUST
         REPORT       LEICESTER LE1 5WW
                      Telephone: 0116 254 1414 Ext. 6536/6546    Lab No.:

UNIT No.:
NAME:


SEX: M          DATE OF BIRTH: 29 years
SPECIMEN: Semen
SITE:
REQUEST:
BY:

   DATE/TIME COLLECTED:        DATE/TIME RECEIVED:
      08.00                       09.00


   Volume      = 4 mls
   Appearance  = Normal
   Sperm Count = no spermatozoa seen
   Motility    = nil
   Morphology  = nil
   Cells       = 5 wcc/ml




   DATE/TIME TELEPHONED:     DATE/TIME REPORTED:     Signature
```

Fig. 9

Pelvic inflammatory disease and genitourinary medicine

1 This photograph (Fig. 12, see also colour plate section) was taken from a 21-year-old single patient.
a. What is the diagnosis?
b. How may this patient have presented?
c. What is the cause of this condition?
d. Where else will you look for similar lesions?
e. What other investigation will you perform on this patient?
f. If untreated, what may it lead to?

2 A 17-year-old is complaining of right upper quadrant abdominal pain and bilateral lower abdominal pain. She is sexually active but is not on any form of contraception. On examination, her temperature is 37.6°C; the right upper quadrant is tender and there is generalized lower abdominal tenderness. Her adnexa are very tender and cervical excitation tenderness is positive on both sides.
a. What is the most likely diagnosis in this patient?
b. What are the two most common causes of this condition?
c. What four investigations would you like to perform on her?
d. Why is she complaining of right upper quadrant pain?
e. What treatment will you offer this patient?

3 A 26-year-old **nulliparous woman underwent surgery and the specimen removed at surgery is shown in Fig. 13** (see also colour plate section).
a. What five symptoms might she have presented with?
b. Which two common organisms may be responsible for the pathology?
c. What additional treatment will you offer her?
d. What is the diagnosis from the specimen?

Hospital

Consultant

Patient's Name   Age 28 years

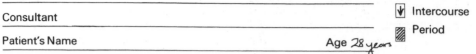

☑ Intercourse

▨ Period

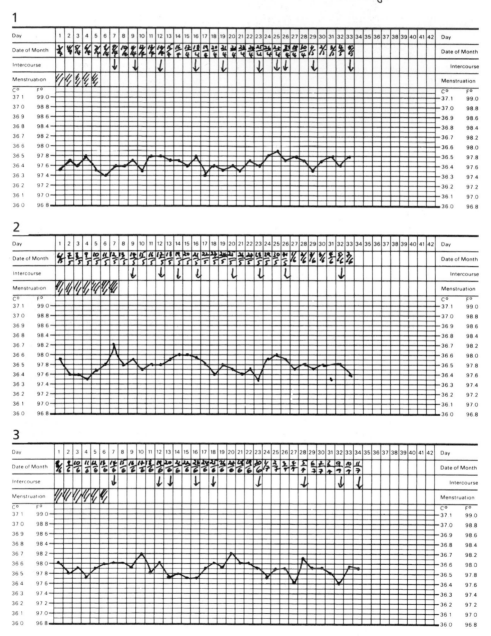

Fig. 10

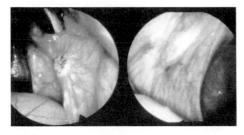

Fig. 11

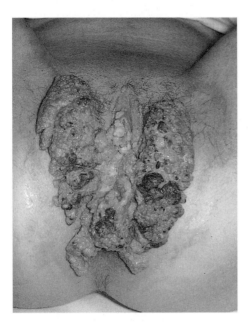

Fig. 12

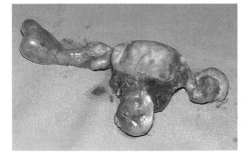

Fig. 13

4 This slide (Fig. 14, see also colour plate section) shows a preparation from a discharge from the urethra of a 22-year-old female student who presented with dysuria.

a. What does the slide show?
b. In which other three ways may she have presented?
c. What treatment will you offer her?
d. What other two steps would you like to take?

5 Miss AF was seen in the genitourinary medicine clinic and a high vaginal swab was obtained from her. Figure 15 (see also colour plate section) was taken from the slide.

a. Identify the organism present in the photograph.
b. In what four ways may the patient have presented?

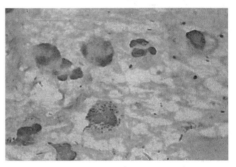

Fig. 14

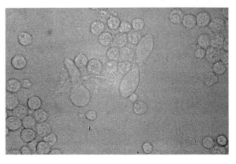

Fig. 15

c. What two signs apart from discharge may she have?

d. What treatment (specify dose and duration) will you offer?

e. What other advice will you offer the patient during treatment?

6 A 31-year-old woman has come to see you for counselling because she has recently had sexual intercourse with a bisexual man.

a. What may be the main reason why she has come to see you?

b. What are the four risk factors for this infection?

c. What is the incubation period of this infection?

d. What may be the initial manifestations of this infection?

e. Which is the virus responsible for the infection?

7 A young girl presented to the family planning clinic for an intrauterine contraceptive device. During pelvic examination, she was found to have small symmetrical ulcers on both labia majora and the vaginal wall. The ulcers were rounded with clearly defined borders and a firm base on palpation.

a. What other clinical sign would you look for?

b. What is the likely diagnosis?

c. What three investigations would you perform to confirm your diagnosis?

d. What treatment would you recommend for her?

e. What complications may arise if she is not treated?

8 A young girl attended the genitourinary medicine clinic and an endocervical swab was reported as showing intracellular Gram-positive diplococci.

a. What is the most likely diagnosis?

b. What symptoms may she present with?

c. What other swabs may you perform on her?

d. What other organisms may you screen for?

e. How will you manage her?

9 The incidence of pelvic inflammatory disease is rising in the UK and worldwide.

a. Identify five risk factors responsible for this trend.

b. Which two forms of contraception are protective against pelvic inflammatory disease?

c. Which four organisms may cause such diseases?

d. Give five symptoms of chronic pelvic inflammatory disease.

10 Mrs BT is a 33- year-old Asian woman who has recently come to settle in England. She presented with vague abdominal pains, irregular periods and infertility. A hysterosalpingogram (Fig. 16) performed as part of her infertility work-up showed 'bead-like' and narrow fallopian tubes with clubbing at the ampulla and calcification in the wall of the tubes.

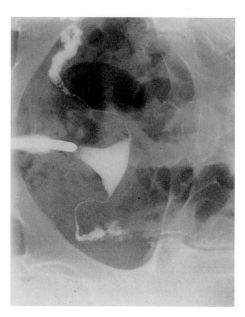

Fig. 16

a. What may be the cause of the tubal pathology?
b. What other three symptoms may she present with?
c. What two investigations will you perform to confirm your diagnosis?
d. What is the likely primary site of this pathology and how did it get to the pelvis?
e. What is the recommended treatment?
f. What is the prognosis of her infertility in the absence of assisted conception methods?

Genital prolapse and urinary incontinence

1 This frequency and volume chart (Fig. 17) was obtained from a 46-year-old woman complaining of involuntary leakage of urine during coughing and aerobics.
a. What other three investigations would you like to perform on her?
b. What is the likely type of incontinence?

c. What four findings from urodynamic investigations will confirm your diagnosis?
d. What treatment options could she have (assuming she has no prolapse)?

2 A 70-year-old nulliparous woman presents with nocturnal enuresis, nocturia, frequency of micturition, urgency and urge incontinence.
a. What is the most likely diagnosis?
b. What would be your differential diagnoses?
c. What three investigations (excluding examination) will you perform on her?
d. What four treatment options are available for her?

3 Mrs White is a 67-year-old widow who has been told that she has a second degree uterine prolapse.
a. What is a second degree uterine prolapse?
b. What four symptoms may she have presented with?
c. What three additional associated pathologies must be excluded on examination?
d. What treatment options may she be offered?

Fig. 17

Name:

Date	Time	Volume in (mls)	Volume out (mls)	Comments
21.12.97	0700		350	
	0800	300 (coffee)		
	0900			
	1000			10.60* wet on sneezing
	1100	250 (coffee)	300	
	1200			
	1300			
	1400		275	
	1500	200 (water)		
	1600			
	1700			16.52* wet on standing up
	1800	200 (tea)	300	
	1900			
	2000			
	2100	250 (coffee)		
	2200		375*	Wet before going to loo

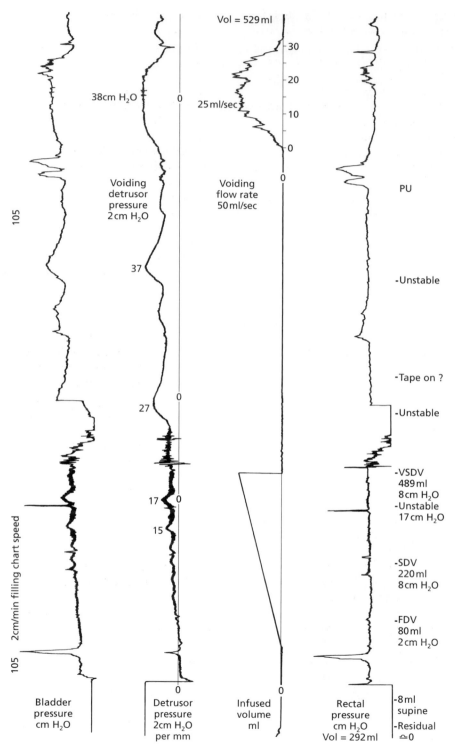

Vol = 529 ml

38cm H₂O

Voiding
detrusor
pressure
2cm H₂O

25 ml/sec

Voiding
flow rate
50 ml/sec

PU

105

37

-Unstable

-Tape on ?

27

-Unstable

2cm/min filling chart speed

17

15

-VSDV
489 ml
8cm H₂O
-Unstable
17cm H₂O

-SDV
220 ml
8cm H₂O

-FDV
80 ml
2cm H₂O

105

Bladder
pressure
cm H₂O

Detrusor
pressure
2cm H₂O
per mm

Infused
volume
ml

Rectal
pressure
cm H₂O
Vol = 292 ml

-8 ml
supine
-Residual
≙0

Fig. 18

4 This cystometry report (Fig. 18) is from a 38-year-old housewife referred by her GP.
a. What is the most likely diagnosis?
b. What other two investigations would you like to perform on her?
c. What four symptoms may she have presented with?
d. What drug treatment would you recommend for her?
e. Give two side-effects of this treatment.

5 A 46-year-old woman underwent a vaginal hysterectomy four weeks ago. Four days after surgery, she has, however, noticed that she constantly wets herself.
a. What is the likely cause of her symptom?
b. How will you confirm this diagnosis?
c. What investigations would you like to perform before offering her treatment?
d. What are long-term complicatons of this condition if untreated?

6 This photograph (Fig. 19, see also colour plate section) was taken from a 70-year-old woman who was seen in the gynaecology clinic.

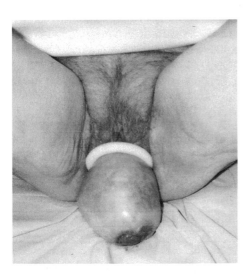

Fig. 19

a. What is the diagnosis?
b. What is the ulcer called?
c. What is the pathophysiology of the ulcer?
d. What must be done to reduce morbidity following surgery?
e. Give four predisposing factors to your diagnosis.

7 Give two complications that may arise from the use of the following instruments.
a. Ring pessary.
b. Shelf pessary.
c. Under what conditions would you use either of them in patients with prolapse?
d. How long should they be left *in situ* and why?

8 A 55-year-old woman with multiple sclerosis has been referred for urogynaecological evaluation because of urinary incontinence, frequency, nocturia, urgency and urge incontinence. At cystometry the intravesical pressure is reported to have risen steadily during filling.
a. What is the most likely diagnosis?
b. What treatment may she be offered?
c. What is the most likely cause of her urinary incontinence?
d. What other investigation should she have?

Family planning and psychosexual medicine

1 A 17-year-old student has been referred to you for emergency postcoital contraception.
a. What two important questions would you like to ask her?
b. What three options are available to her?
c. What instructions will you give her about the tablets?

d. How may antibiotics affect the efficacy of the tablets?

e. What further advice must you give her?

2 Figure 20 shows a method of contraception.

a. What is it called?

b. List four contraindications for its use.

c. Give three side-effects of this method of contraception.

d. What instructions will you give a patient after inserting this device?

3 A patient has reported to you because she cannot feel the string of her intrauterine contraceptive device which you inserted six months ago.

a. What may be responsible for this?

b. Which four methods may be useful in locating the device?

c. If the device has migrated into the peritoneal cavity, what would be your plan of management?

d. When is perforation likely to occur and why?

4 A family planning clinic practice nurse has just referred a patient to you with an intrauterine contraceptive device *in situ*, six weeks' amenorrhoea and a viable intrauterine pregnancy on scan.

a. What two options are available for her management?

b. What complications may arise for each of the options above?

5 Figure 21 shows a photograph of a method of contraception.

a. What is the form of contraception?

b. How long is it expected to last?

c. What is the active compound in this method of contraception?

d. Name four common side-effects of this method of contraception.

e. Give two contraindications to the use of this method of contraception.

f. What is the failure rate of this method of contraception?

6 A 32-year-old woman who has completed her family and is currently on the combined oral contraceptive pill wishes to be referred for sterilization. She would, however, like more information before she decides on the procedure.

a. What is the failure rate of the method?

b. How may the fallopian tubes be approached?

c. What two devices may be used for tubal occlusion?

d. Are there any other complications of the procedure?

e. What other information would you like to offer her?

7 Figure 22 shows five methods of contraception. Identify each of them and give a contraindication for its use and its failure rate.

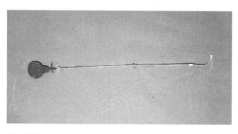

Fig. 20

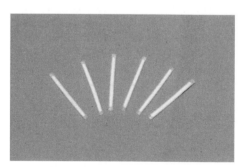

Fig. 21

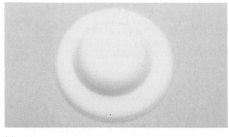

(a)

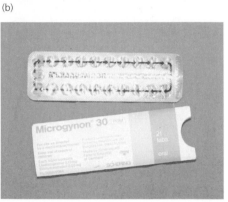

(b)

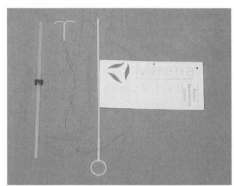

(c)

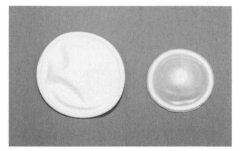

(d)

Fig. 22

(e)

8 A young couple are seeking counselling because they are experiencing sexual dysfunction.
a. List five types of female sexual dysfunction.
b. List four types of male sexual dysfunction.
c. In taking the history from the couple, what five factors will you be addressing?
d. What four methods of treating male erectile dysfunction are available?

Menopause

1 A 34-year-old woman with secondary amenorrhoea of 18 months' duration has just attended the gynaecology clinic for consultation. An ultrasound scan of the pelvis revealed a small uterus and no adnexal masses. Her hormone profile is shown in Fig. 23.
a. What is the most likely diagnosis?
b. What other six symptoms may she have presented with?

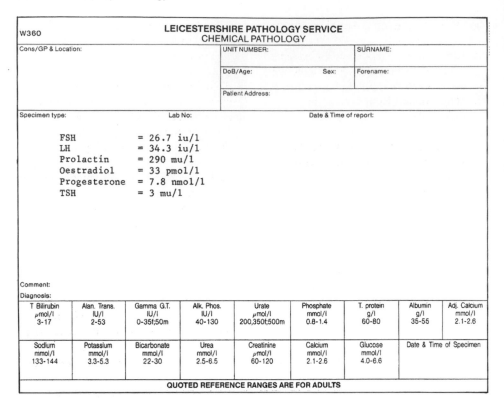

W360		LEICESTERSHIRE PATHOLOGY SERVICE							
		CHEMICAL PATHOLOGY							

Cons/GP & Location:

UNIT NUMBER: SURNAME:

DoB/Age: Sex: Forename:

Patient Address:

Specimen type: Lab No: Date & Time of report:

```
FSH          = 26.7 iu/l
LH           = 34.3 iu/l
Prolactin    = 290 mu/l
Oestradiol   = 33 pmol/l
Progesterone = 7.8 nmol/l
TSH          = 3 mu/l
```

Comment:

Diagnosis:

T Bilirubin μmol/l 3-17	Alan. Trans. IU/l 2-53	Gamma G.T. IU/l 0-35f;50m	Alk. Phos. IU/l 40-130	Urate μmol/l 200,350f;500m	Phosphate mmol/l 0.8-1.4	T. protein g/l 60-80	Albumin g/l 35-55	Adj. Calcium mmol/l 2.1-2.6

Sodium mmol/l 133-144	Potassium mmol/l 3.3-5.3	Bicarbonate mmol/l 22-30	Urea mmol/l 2.5-6.5	Creatinine μmol/l 60-120	Calcium mmol/l 2.1-2.6	Glucose mmol/l 4.0-6.6	Date & Time of Specimen	

QUOTED REFERENCE RANGES ARE FOR ADULTS

Fig. 23

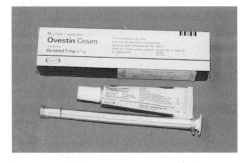

Fig. 24

c. What treatment will you offer her?
d. What are three main benefits of this treatment?

2 A 42-year-old teacher has just had a total abdominal hysterectomy and bilateral salpingo-ophorectomy. She has been discharged home and has come to see you with some questions about hormone replacement therapy (HRT).
a. What five diseases/disabilities may HRT prevent?
b. By which three methods can she take her HRT?
c. List four contraindications to HRT.
d. How long will she have to go on HRT?

3 Identify the drug shown in Fig. 24.
a. What is the name of the drug?
b. Give four indications for its use.
c. What are the complications of this drug?
d. Name two absolute contraindications for its use.

4 A 78-year-old woman presents with a two-month history of post-menopausal bleeding which has been irregular and heavy.
a. What are the two most common causes of post-menopausal bleeding?

b. What investigations would you like to perform on her?

c. If the histology report shows benign glandular hyperplasia, what treatment options will be available?

d. When might a hysterectomy be indicated?

5 A young and fit mother of three has come to see you for some information about the menopause.

a. What are the risk factors for osteoporosis?

b. What investigation may be predictive?

c. What preventative measures can be taken?

d. What type of HRT may improve libido?

e. What is the risk of developing deep venous thrombosis and breast cancer on HRT?

6 Mrs OAT is 52 years old and has had a benign breast lump excised recently. She is requesting HRT.

a. Are benign breast lumps a contraindication to HRT?

b. She would like to take oestrogens alone but would like to know the risks. What are they?

c. How may some of the side-effects of oestrogen replacement therapy be overcome?

d. How may some of the complications of HRT be prevented?

Gynaecological tumours (benign and malignant)

1 A 21-year-old woman's cervical smear is reported as follows: 'Mild dyskaryosis present'.

a. What three important points would you emphasize during counselling?

b. Which three smear abnormalities would merit immediate referral for colposcopy following a single report?

c. What advice would you offer a young woman who has undergone colposcopy with loop excision of the transformation zone (LLETZ) to treat cervical intraepithelial neoplasia?

2 A cold knife cone biopsy is rarely performed nowadays in the treatment of cervical intraepithelial neoplasia.

a. Under what conditions would the performance of a cone biopsy be necessary?

b. What are four possible complications of cold knife cone biopsy?

c. What are the two disadvantages of cone biopsy over LLETZ?

d. What three other methods of local treatment of cervical intraepithelial neoplasia are available?

3 A 35-year-old woman presented with intermenstrual and post-coital bleeding. A speculum examination revealed an obvious lesion (Fig. 25, see also colour plate section). She had a normal smear one year ago.

a. What is the mosy likely diagnosis?

b. How would you confirm your diagnosis?

c. What procedures must be performed to satisfactorily stage the disease?

d. What four relevant investigations might you perform on her?

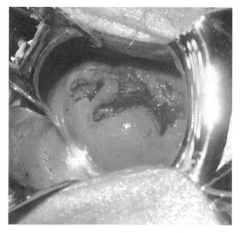

Fig. 25

e. What two treatment options may she be offered?

4 A 69-year-old woman with a past history of breast cancer has been taking Tamoxifen for five years. She presents with post-menopausal bleeding.
a. What three important investigations might you perform on her?
b. What three pathological abnormalities may be present?
c. What two treatment options are available for this range of abnormalities?

5 Miss K, aged 32 years, has recently lost her sister aged 38 years to ovarian cancer. Her mother died of an intra-abdominal malignancy which turned out to be ovarian cancer. She is unmarried and uses barrier methods of contraception.
a. How would you counsel her about her risk of developing ovarian cancer?
b. What three factors could reduce her risk?
c. What screening methods are currently available?
d. What prophylactic measures can be offered to Miss K?

6 A 25-year-old woman in her first pregnancy reports vaginal bleeding at 10 weeks' gestation. On examination, the uterus is enlarged to the equivalent of 14 weeks and an ultrasound scan shows a 'snow storm' appearance with the absence of a fetus.
a. What is the likely diagnosis?
b. What preoperative investigations should be performed?
c. What is the primary management of the condition?
d. What follow-up is indicated?

7 A 45-year-old patient presents with a pelvic mass equivalent to a 16-week pregnancy. An ultrasound scan report is as follows: 'There is a multicystic mass with solid areas arising from the pelvis. The uterus is normal in size, but neither ovary can be identified. There is a moderate amount of ascites'.
a. What is the most likely diagnosis?
b. What additional symptoms may she have presented with?
c. What preoperative investigations would be considered useful in this case?
d. At surgery she is said to have stage III disease. What does this mean?

8 A 64-year-old woman presented with weight loss, anorexia and an offensive vaginal discharge. Examination revealed a tumour involving the cervix and extending down into the upper two-thirds of the vagina. The pelvis appear fixed. A biopsy showed it to be a squamous cell carcinoma.
a. What stage is this disease?
b. What two treatment options are available for this patient?
c. The oncologist has decided to offer her radiotherapy. What three complications may be experienced during treatment?
d. What are the six possible long-term complications of radiotherapy?

9 A 65-year-old obese diabetic woman presented with post-menopausal bleeding. Hysteroscopy showed an irregular polypoid tumour at the fundus, biopsy of which revealed a poorly differentiated (grade 3) adenocarcinoma consistent with a primary endometrial carcinoma.
a. What five factors are associated with an increased risk of endometrial carcinoma?
b. What is the primary treatment of choice in this patient?
c. Which alternate method of treatment may she have, assuming she is not fit for surgery?
d. The histology report following surgery shows a poorly differentiated (grade 3) endometrial adenocarcinoma, invading into the outer half of the myometrium.

The peritoneal cytology and lymph node sampling are negative for metastatic tumour. What FIGO stage is the disease?

e. Which are the two poor prognostic factors in this case.

10 A 29-year-old woman with no children has been diagnosed as having stage Ib carcinoma of the cervix. She has been admitted to undergo a Wertheim's hysterectomy and pelvic lymph node dissection. She has a few questions for you.

a. What is stage Ib carcinoma of the cervix?
b. What does the operation entail?
c. She is worried about the postoperative complications – both short and long term. What are four possible short-term complications?
d. What are the long-term complications (give three)?
e. Will adjuvant therapy be necessary and what will this be? What will affect prognosis in this patient?

11 A 21-year-old student nurse is admitted as an emergency with acute-onset intermittent right iliac fossa and loin pain. Her last period was one week ago and a pregnancy test was negative. On examination, she has rebound tenderness in the lower abdomen. On vaginal examination, there is a right adnexal mass which on scan is shown to measure 6 × 8 cm and is partly solid and partly cystic. The uterus and the left ovary are described as normal.

a. What is the likely diagnosis?
b. What are your differential diagnoses?
c. Is there any other non-invasive investigation that may confirm your diagnosis?
d. What is the definitive management?
e. What are dermoid cysts of the ovary?

12 Mrs DT is a 64-year-old diabetic who
is complaining of post-menopausal bleeding.

a. How would you investigate her?
b. Histology of the endometrium reveals a grade 3 endometrial adenocarcinoma. What is the primary treatment of choice in this patient?
c. What other primary therapies might be considered.
d. What four poor prognostic features would indicate that adjuvant therapy might be useful in this patient?

13 A 75-year-old woman presents with vague abdominal symptoms. Over the past two months she has noticed increasing swelling of her abdomen. On examination she has a very distended abdomen with shifting dullness.

a. What initial investigations would you consider?
b. The investigations reveal that advanced ovarian cancer is the most likely diagnosis and laparotomy is planned. How would you counsel the patient preoperatively regarding the operative procedure?
c. Optimum debulking has been performed. What adjuvant therapy will be considered?
d. What is the prognosis if it is stage IV disease?

14 Mrs Turner, a 37-year-old nulliparous woman, is complaining of heavy and regular periods. She has also noticed a mass in her lower abdomen. She only experiences pain during the heavy days of her periods. On examination, there is an abdominal mass the size of 16 weeks' gestation arising from the pelvis. The mass is described as irregular and firm in consistency.

a. What is the most likely diagnosis?
b. How would you confirm your diagnosis?
c. What other signs or symptoms may the patient have presented with?

d. What surgical treatment would you offer Mrs Turner in view of the fact that she wishes to have children?
e. What is the danger of this operation?
f. How may the risk of this complication occurring be reduced?

15 This tumour (Fig. 26, see also colour plate section) was taken from a 39-year-old woman at surgery.
a. What is the diagnosis?
b. How may she have presented?
c. Give four complications of this condition.
d. What is the alternative method of treatment in this case?

16 A 30-year-old schoolteacher has presented to her GP with chest pain. A chest X-ray showed a right-sided pleural effusion.
a. Which benign gynaecological pathology will present with pleural effusion?
b. What is this clinical combination called?
c. How can this diagnosis be confirmed?
d. What other two clinical signs may be present?
e. What is the treatment of choice?

17 A histology report from a 42-year-old woman presenting with irregular and heavy periods is shown in Fig. 27 (see also colour plate section).
a. What is the diagnosis?

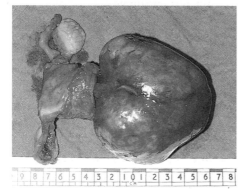

Fig. 26

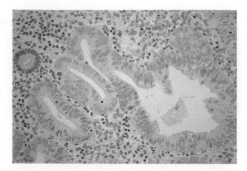

Fig. 27

b. What three factors could predispose to this condition?
c. What is the risk of this condition if it is left untreated?
d. What is the primary treatment you would recommend to the woman?
e. Give three conditions in which this pathology may be found.

18 Mrs Peters has observed that her breasts are getting smaller and her periods have become very infrequent and scanty. She has had a hormone profile and the results are shown in Fig. 28.
a. What is Mrs Peters experiencing?
b. What may be responsible for this condition?
c. How would you make a diagnosis?
d. What other three symptoms may the patient present with?
e. What treatment will you offer her?

19 The following slides in Fig. 29 (see also colour plate section) show various pathologies. Identify each of them.

20 A 17-year-old girl presented with an abdominal mass which was confirmed to be ovarian in origin on scan. Serum alpha-fetoprotein levels were significantly high.
a. What is the likely diagnosis in this case?
b. List four other types of malignant germ cell tumours.
c. What is the treatment of choice in this

W360	LEICESTERSHIRE PATHOLOGY SERVICE		
	CHEMICAL PATHOLOGY		

Cons/GP & Location:	UNIT NUMBER:		SURNAME:
	DoB/Age: 24.1.70	Sex: F	Forename:
	Patient Address:		

Specimen type:	Lab No:	Date & Time of report:

```
FSH              = 5.7 iu/l
LH               = 6.2 iu/l
Androstenedione  = 27.4 nmol/l
Testosterone     = 3.7 nmol/l
Oestradiol       = 280 pmol/l
Progesterone     = 10.7 nmol/l
TSH              = 2.7 mu/l
```

Comment:

Diagnosis:

T Bilirubin μmol/l 3-17	Alan. Trans. IU/l 2-53	Gamma G.T. IU/l 0-35f;50m	Alk. Phos. IU/l 40-130	Urate μmol/l 200,350f;500m	Phosphate mmol/l 0.8-1.4	T. protein g/l 60-80	Albumin g/l 35-55	Adj. Calcium mmol/l 2.1-2.6

Sodium mmol/l 133-144	Potassium mmol/l 3.3-5.3	Bicarbonate mmol/l 22-30	Urea mmol/l 2.5-6.5	Creatinine μmol/l 60-120	Calcium mmol/l 2.1-2.6	Glucose mmol/l 4.0-6.6	Date & Time of Specimen

QUOTED REFERENCE RANGES ARE FOR ADULTS

Fig. 28

patient if the tumour is confined to one ovary?

d. How will follow-up be monitored?

Vulvar disorders

1 Figure 30 (see also colour plate section) was taken from a 75-year-old woman who presented with a blood-stained discharge.

a. What is the likely diagnosis?

b. Name three histological types of this condition.

c. What three underlying aetiological factors may predispose to the development of this condition?

d. What is likely to be the management of this woman?

e. What is the prognosis?

2 A 74-year-old woman presents with pruritus vulvae. Examination reveals an atrophic-looking vulva with mild leukoplakia. Vulva biopsy reveals lichen sclerosus.

a. What four symptoms may she also present with?

b. To which class of conditions of the vulva does it belong?

c. What three typical signs may be demonstrated in this patient?

d. What three treatment options might you recommend?

e. Has surgery any role in the management of this condition?

f. What is the long-term prognosis of this condition?

3 Figure 31 (see also colour plate section) was taken from a 35-year-old woman.

a. What symptoms may she have presented with?

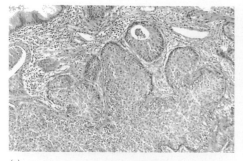

(a)

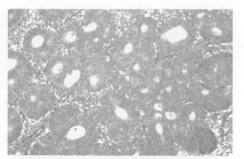

(b)

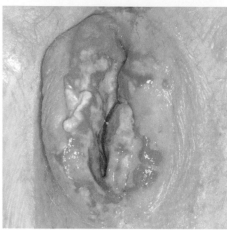

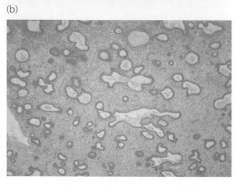

(d)

(c)

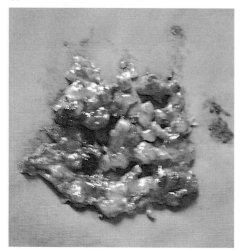

(e)

Fig. 29

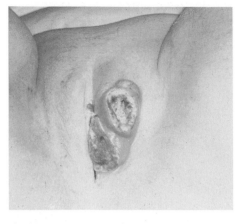

Fig. 30

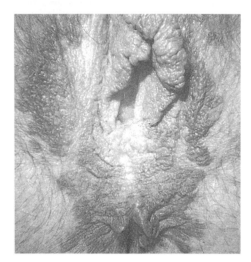

Fig. 31

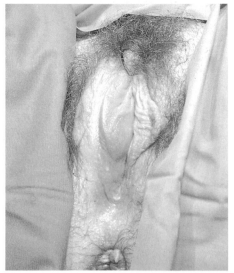

Fig. 32

a. What is the likely diagnosis?
b. What are the four most common organisms for this condition?
c. What four symptoms may the patient present with?
d. What is the treatment of choice?

5 Figure 33 (see also colour plate section) was obtained from a young girl in the gynaecology out-patient department.
a. What is the likely diagnosis?
b. What symptoms may she have presented with?

b. What are the most likely differential diagnoses?
c. What three investigations should be performed on her?
d. By which four methods may the patient be managed?
e. How should the patient be followed-up?

4 Figure 32 (see also colour plate section) is taken from a young sexually active girl presenting as an emergency.

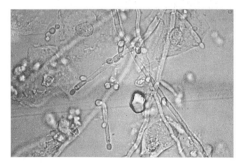

Fig. 33

c. What signs may be present on examination?
d. What factors predispose to the occurrence of this infection?
e. What is the treatment for this patient?

6 This lesion (Fig. 34, see also colour plate section) was found in an 80-year-old woman who was referred by her GP as an emergency. She had had it for over 10 years.
a. What are your differential diagnoses?
b. What is the ulcer on top of the lesion called?
c. What investigation may she have to confirm the diagnosis?
d. What treatment options are available?

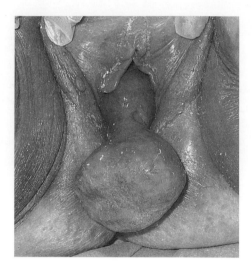

Fig. 34

Gynaecological surgery

1 A nulliparous women in her late twenties presented with regular and heavy periods. She is married and would like to have children. A full blood count performed on her is shown in Fig. 35.
a. What are the abnormalities in the report?
b. What further investigations would you like to perform on her?
c. What would be your initial line of management assuming that a pelvic examination was normal?
d. What other two treatment options might you offer her if the above fail?
e. If in addition, she experiences severe pain during menstruation and her uterus is described as bulky during pelvic examination but ultrasound scan failed to demonstrate any fibroids, what would be the most likely diagnosis?

2 The vital signs chart (Fig. 36) is that of a 56-year-old woman who had a total abdominal hysterectomy four days ago.
a. What symptoms may she present with?

b. What are the common causes of her symptoms?
c. What five investigations will you perform to confirm your diagnosis?
d. What would be your initial management plan if she has an infected pelvic haematoma?

3 A 50-year-old woman who had a vaginal hysterectomy six hours ago has not been able to pass any urine since returning from theatre. She has, however, had 3 litres of intravenous fluids. She has a catheter *in situ*.
a. What clinical symptoms should be enquired about?
b. What clinical signs would assist you in making a diagnosis?
c. What are the three possible causes of her problem?
d. What would be your immediate management of these three conditions?

4 The instruments in Fig. 37 are numbered a to j. They are commonly used in the gynaecology outpatient theatre. Identify each of the instruments and give an indication for its use.

LEICESTERSHIRE HAEMATOLOGY SERVICE					Tel. ext: LRI 6530: LGH 4566: GGH 3575				

Consultant + Patient Loc.				SURNAME			FORENAME		
or GP Name + address				SEX F	DOB/AGE 27 years		HOSPITAL No.	LABORATORY No.	

Differential	Neutrophils	Lymphocytes	Monocytes	Eosinophils	Basophils	Atypical Lymph.	Metamyelo	Myelocytes	Pro. Mye	Blasts
WBC % x 10⁹/1	76.0 6.84	16.9 1.52	4.9 0.44	1.8 0.16	0.4 0.004					
% Adults Normal Range ABS	40-75 2.0-7.5	20-45 1.5-4.0	2-10 0.2-0.8	1-6 0.04-0.4	1 or less 0.01-0.1					

Machine Differential	Granulocytes	Lymphocytes	Mononuclears	WHITE CELL COMMENT						
WBC %	%	%	%							

Hb	RBC	HCT	MCV	MCH	Reticulocytes	WBC	Platelets	P.V.	Date of Sample 19.06.1997
M 13.5-18.0 F 11.5-16.5	M 4.5-6.5 F 3.9-5.6	M 0.4-0.54 F 0.37-0.47	80-99	27 - 32	0 - 2	4 - 11	150-400	1.5-1.72	Date Reported 19.06.1997
9.2 g/dl	4.7 x 10¹²/1	0.292	70.1 fl	22.4 pg	%	7.4 x 10⁹/1	750 x 10⁹/1	cp	Run Page of

Fig. 35

Interactive questions

COUNSELLING QUESTIONS

The following questions may be posed at an interactive station where there is a role-player or where there is an examiner playing the role of a patient. In the absence of the role-player, hints will be provided on the answers. It is advisable for candidates to practice these scenarios by casting their nets as wide as possible.

1 Mrs Peters is a 27-year-old mother of two who would like to be sterilized. She has come to see you for counselling about sterilization.
In counselling this young woman, it is important to explain the implications of the procedure. The failure rate of sterilization must be quoted and explained in language that is easy to comprehend. Most experts quote a failure rate of 1 : 300. The candidate must explain that failure means that Mrs Peters may become pregnant. The risk of an ectopic pregnancy if there is failure should be mentioned and reasons for this offered. Is the patient aware that there are other methods of contraception like the intrauterine contraceptive device, Norplant and vasectomy. Have the couple discussed these alternatives? Although sterilization is not irreversible *per se*, most people consider the procedure irreversible and this point should be mentioned. Finally, the means by which sterilization is performed should be explained (by laparoscopy with a proviso of resorting to a minilaparotomy

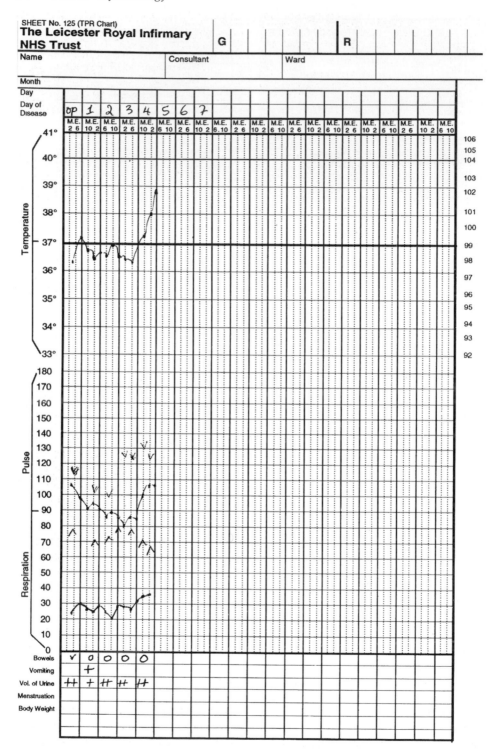

Fig. 36

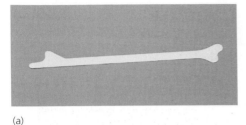

(a)

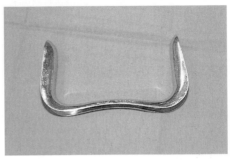

(b)

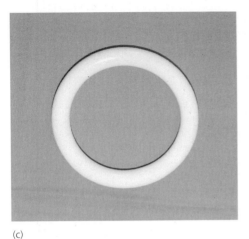

(c)

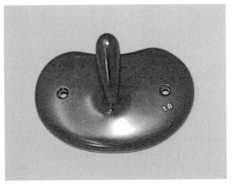

(d)

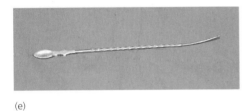

(e)

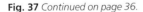

(f)

Fig. 37 *Continued on page 36.*

where laparoscopy is difficult). It may be prudent to mention that there is a long waiting list and that in the interim, the patient must use an effective means of contraception. The candidate must not forget to discuss the type of anaesthesia the patient may have, the consequences of

coming off the pill on menstruation (if the patient is on the pill) and the time it will take to return to work.

2 You performed a routine cervical smear on a young girl six weeks ago and she has come back for the results. The report reads

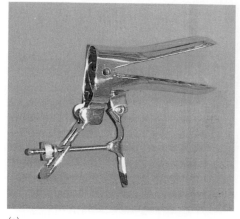

(g)

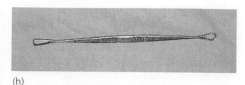

(h)

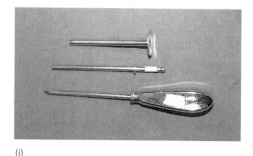

(i)

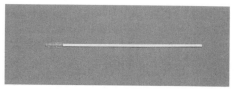

(j)

Fig. 37 *(Continued)*

'moderate dyskaryosis'. Counsel her about the result and further management.
The most important point is that the patient is reassured that she does *not* have cancer. She has an abnormal smear (abnormal cells which may lead to cancer after 10–15 years if untreated) and therefore needs further evaluation. She will need referral for colposcopy where the cervix will be examined under a special microscope and further treatment may be offered if necessary. In most cases, a definitive treatment is offered at this visit. Such a treatment is adequate in most cases. She would, however, require follow-up smears for at least five years. The treatment she receives is unlikely to affect either her future reproductive potential or her

menstrual cycle. The candidate must understand the apprehension that the patient may have and must try to be very reassuring. The language used must be free of technical terms.

3 A 31-year-old woman who recently had a miscarriage completed by an evacuation of the uterus has come back to see you because the histology report of the products of conception concluded that '. . . the findings are consistent with a complete hydatidiform mole'. Could you discuss these findings and her subsequent management.
This is a difficult problem because there are no equivalent lay terms for molar pregnancy. The candidate must therefore

try to explain as much as possible using diagrams and using the placenta (afterbirth) as an analogy. The important message is that the patient does not have a malignancy. There is, however, the need for follow-up because of the risk of progression to persistent disease and occasionally malignancy. The advantage of follow-up is that those minority cases that will progress to malignancy when identified early will in most cases be completely cured without any deleterious effects on their reproductive ability. The follow-up will be by serial urine and blood tests which are performed in three centres in the UK (namely Sheffield, Dundee and Charing Cross, London – the candidates must be aware of the centre in their region). Pregnancy must be avoided for at least six months following the miscarriage as it may interfere with the follow-up. The intrauterine contraceptive device must be avoided. The combined oral contraceptive pill is also to be avoided until the β-HCG levels have returned to normal. The method of contraception to be offered at this stage is a barrier method of contraception with a spermicidal cream. Following each subsequent pregnancy, she must also be followed-up very closely.

4 Following surgery for a right ectopic gestation, a young girl is about to go home. What advice will you give her?
The recurrence risk following an ectopic gestation is 10 times that in the general population. The patient must therefore report to her GP as soon as she misses a period. This is so that any recurrent ectopic pregnancy can be identified early and the tube saved if possible. The successful pregnancy rate following conservative surgery on the tube is much higher than that following IVF. The candidate must advise the patient about the most appropriate method of contraception. The intrauterine contraceptive device and

progestogen-only contraceptives should be avoided. The combined oral contraceptive pill is an effective method.

5 A 42-year-old woman who has recently had a total abdominal hysterectomy and bilateral salpingo-ophorectomy would like to go on HRT. She, however, would like to be advised.
The counselling should highlight the advantages of having HRT for a woman of this age. The rare side-effects of HRT such as breast cancer and deep venous thrombosis should be mentioned but the candidate must emphasize that the patient is more likely to die from complications of not taking HRT than she is from taking them. The need for regular breast examinations should be mentioned. For the HRT to be effective, it has to be taken for at least 10 years to protect against osteoporosis and cardiovascular disorders. Since the patient has no uterus, she would only require oestrogens which can be taken orally, as implants or as transdermal patches/gels.

6 A student at the university has come to see you about the combined oral contraceptive pill. She does not have any contraindications and you have prescribed Microgynon 30 for her. What advice will you give her?
The issues that require addressing here are when to start the pill, how to take it, what to do when pills are missed and the effect of drugs and diarrhoea on the efficacy of the pill. Most practitioners would advise that the pills are started within the first five days of menstruation. When taking antibiotics and other drugs such as griseofulvin and antiepileptics, it must be remembered that the efficacy of the pill is compromised. The patient must therefore take extra precautions and similarly when she has diarrhoea. The seven-day rule must be explained and the student encouraged to ask questions.

7 This 22-year-old has come to see you for emergency contraception. What advice will you give her?

This form of contraception is only effective if taken within the prescribed time. It is therefore important to establish why she wants it. It may be that she is planning to have intercourse in which case condoms and a spermicidal cream may be offered. If, however, it is because she has had unprotected sexual intercourse, then the time of intercourse must be established. The first date of her last menstrual period must also be ascertained. Having established these facts, the options available must be discussed. The most obvious one will be the PC4, two tablets of which must be taken immediately and the other two taken after 12 hours. If there is any vomiting then the tablets must be retaken. These are only effective if taken within 72 hours of sexual intercourse. The other option is the intrauterine contraceptive device. This can be effective up to five days after sexual intercourse. Finally, a more effective contraceptive method must be discussed and the patient advised as to what to do should the emergency contraception not work. The failure rate is 1–5% depending on the stage of the menstrual cycle during which the sexual intercourse took place.

8 This 32-year-old woman attended the gynaecology clinic with post-coital bleeding and has returned for the results of a punch biopsy which was taken in the clinic. The histology reads 'well differentiated squamous cell carcinoma of the cervix'. Could you counsel her about the diagnosis and treatment.

9 A mother has brought her daughter to you because she has primary amenorrhoea. Investigations which you have organized indicate that she has testicular feminizing syndrome. Her karyotype is 46XY and she has gonads in her groin. She is very anxious and would like your advice before she goes back to see the surgeon.

10 A young woman has just been told by her boyfriend that he is HIV positive. He had in fact been an intravenous drug user in the past but has not had any drugs for the past 12 months. She has come to see you about counselling on whether she should have an HIV test or not.

11 A 27-year-old nulliparous woman with a diagnosis of polycystic ovarian syndrome requires clomiphene citrate for induction of ovulation. Advice her on the treatment and its complications.

12 A very worried woman has come to see you for advice about the implications of polycystic ovarian syndrome. She has been told that it may affect her fertility and her future health.

HISTORY QUESTIONS

1 This 58-year-old woman is presenting with urinary incontinence. Take a relevant history and formulate a differential diagnosis.

2 This young girl aged 20 years old is complaining of abdominal pain and vaginal bleeding. Take a relevant history and establish your most likely diagnosis.

3 Mrs Brown has had period problems for the past six years. She is 30 years old, nulliparous, married and is not on any form of contraception. Take a relevant history and give your differential diagnoses.

4 A couple married for four years have been trying for a baby for two years unsuccessfully. Take a relevant history and

suggest the most likely explanation for the infertility.

5 Cynthia has been told that she has carcinoma of the cervix stage IIa. Could you answer the few questions she has for you?
a. What is carcinoma of the cervix stage IIa?
b. What investigations would be performed on her?
c. What are the different types of treatment that she could be offered?

d. What complications may arise from these different methods of treatment.

POSSIBLE TASKS QUESTIONS

1 Perform a cervical smear from a model patient.
2 Perform a high vaginal, endocervical or urethral swabs from a model patient with vaginal discharge or symptoms of pelvic inflammatory disease.

ANSWERS

Menstrual disorders

Question 1
a. Asherman's syndrome (uterine synechae).
b. Hysteroscopy.
   Hysterosalpingography.
c. Hysteroscopic division of the adhesions/insertion of an intrauterine contraceptive device following the division of the adhesions and continuous oestrogens to promote endometrial growth.
d. Spontaneous miscarriage.
   Recurrent miscarriage.
   Preterm labour.
   Placenta accreta leading to postpastum haemorrhage.

Question 2
a. Diagnostic therapy with luteinising hormone releasing hormone (LHRH) analogues.
b. Swelling of the legs and fingers.
   Bloated feeling of the abdomen and breasts.
   Greasy skin and acne.
   Headaches.
   Dizziness.
   Palpitations.
   Breast tenderness.
   Changes in bowel and bladder function.
   Mood swings.
c. Oestrogens.
   Progestogens.
   Evening primrose (vitamin E) and pyridoxine.
   Combined oral contraceptive pill.
   Danazol.
   LHRH analogues.
   Placebo.
d. The risk of postpartum depression is greater than 30%.

e. Thirty to 40% of women with premenstrual syndrome (PMS) have mothers who suffer from PMS.

Question 3
a. Full blood count.
   Thyroid function tests.
   Coagulation screening.
b. Menorrhagia.
c. Mefenamic acid.
   Combined oral contraceptive pill.
   Tranexamic acid during menstruation.
   Danazol continuously.
   Progestogen-containing intrauterine contraceptive device (Mirena).
d. Endometrial ablation or resection.
   Hysterectomy (with conservation of the ovaries).

Question 4
a. Turner's syndrome.
b. Short stature.
   Webbed neck.
   Widely spaced nipples.
   Absent secondary sexual characteristics.
   Coarctation of the aorta.
   Wide carrying angle on the upper limbs.
c. Hypoplastic uterus.
   Streaked gonads.
d. Combined oestrogen and progestogen to prevent osteoporosis and cardiovascular disease and to stimulate secondary sexual characteristics and uterine development.
e. She will be infertile but with embryo donation, she may be able to achieve a pregnancy.

Question 5
a. Ultrasound scan.
   Hysteroscopy.

Endometrial biopsy.
b. Dysfunctional uterine bleeding.
c. Cyclical progestogens preferably combined with tranexamic acid.
d. Total abdominal hysterectomy and bilateral salpingo-ophorectomy because the risk of progression to malignancy is about 45%.

Question 6
a. Haematocolpos.
b. Cyclical lower abdominal pain.
   Urinary frequency.
   Urinary retention.
   Lower abdominal mass.
   Apareunia (unsuccessful sexual intercourse).
c. Ultrasound scan of the renal system.
   Intravenous urogram.
d. Incision under general anaesthesia.
e. 46XX.

Question 7
a. Karyotype.
   Urea and electrolytes.
   Examination of the groins for masses.
   Serum 17-alpha-hydroxyprogesterone.
   Plasma testosterone.
b. Correction of any electrolyte imbalance if there is congenital adrenal hyperplasia of the salt-losing type.
c. Congenital adrenal hyperplasia.
d. Autosomal recessive.
e. Steroid maintenance.
   Clitoridectomy at 2–3 years of age.

Early pregnancy disorders

Question 1
a. Hyperemesis gravidarum.
b. Hyperthyroidism.
   Multiple pregnancy.
   Molar pregnancy.
   Urinary tract infections.
c. Urea and electrolytes.
   Ultrasound scan.
   Liver function test.

Urine microscopy and culture.
Thyroid function test.
d. Jaundice.
   Renal failure from electrolyte imbalance.
   Kosakov's syndrome.
   Wernicke's encephalopathy.
   Death.

Question 2
a. Septic incomplete abortion.
b. Tachycardia.
   Lower abdominal tenderness.
   Pelvic tenderness.
c. Full blood count.
   Blood culture.
   Group and save serum.
   Swabs (endocervical and high vaginal) for microscopy/culture/sensitivity.
   Ultrasound scan.
d. Intravenous antibiotics.
   Evacuation of the uterus.
e. Salpingitis which may lead to a tubo-ovarian abscess.
   Septicaemia/septic shock.
   Renal failure.
   Disseminated intravascular coagulation.
   Chronic pelvic inflammatory disease.
   Infertility.
f. *Chlamydia trachomatis.*
   Neisseria gonorrhoeae.
   Escherichia coli.
   Bacteroides fragilis.
   Streptococcus (haemolytic and non-haemolytic).
   Staphylococcus aureus.
   Clostridium welchii.

Question 3
a. Threatened miscarriage.
   Missed abortion.
b. Ultrasound scan. For missed abortion: gestational sac with or without fetus but no fetal heart beat present. For threatened miscarriage: gestational sac and fetal heart beat present.
c. Blood group. If rhesus-negative, she

will require an intramuscular injection of anti-D (250 IU).

d. Missed abortion: evacuation (surgical or medical).
Threatened abortion: reassurance and rest at home.

Question 4

a. Pallor, tachycardia, hypotension, abdominal tenderness, guarding, rebound, tenderness in the fornices, fullness in the pouch of Douglas, open os, blood clots in the vagina.

b. Full blood count.
Group and save.
Kleihauer Betke.
Pelvic ultrasound.
β-HCG.
Diagnostic laparoscopy.

c. Ectopic pregnancy.
Threatened miscarriage.
Incomplete miscarriage.
Complete miscarriage.

d. Threatened miscarriage: bed rest at home or in hospital.
Incomplete miscarriage: ERPC.
Ectopic pregnancy: surgery (salpingectomy or salpingostomy) or medical treatment (for example with methotrexate).
Complete miscarriage: reassurance.

Question 5

a. Ectopic gestation.

b. Pelvic inflammatory disease.
In vitro fertilization and embryo transfer (IVF-ET).
Gamete intrafallopian transfer (GIFT).
Tubal surgery: sterilization or reversal of sterilization.
Previous ectopic gestation.

c. Ultrasound scan.
Diagnostic laparoscopy.

d. Recurrence risk is 10%.
Report if any periods are missed.
Avoid the use of intrauterine contraceptive devices and progestogen-only pills.

Question 6

a. Surgical termination (suction evacuation) under general anaesthesia.
Medical termination with a combination of antiprogestogens and prostaglandins.

b. Suction termination of first trimester pregnancies is not associated with an increased risk of subfertility.

c. Blood group.
Endocervical swab for *Chlamydia*.

d. To use acceptable and effective contraception.

Question 7

a. Hydatidiform mole.

b. Exaggerated symptoms of pregnancy, e.g. excessive vomiting.
Vaginal bleeding.
Passage of vesicles (small grapes).

c. Uterus large for dates.
Absent fetal heart beat on scan.
Raised blood pressure/proteinuria.
Signs of thyrotoxicosis.

d. Registration with a regional centre.
Follow-up by serial β-HCG.
Defer future pregnancy for at least six months.

e. Early identification of choriocarcinoma.
Identification of persistent trophoblastic disease.

Question 8

a. Ectopic gestation.
Torted ovarian cyst.
Haemorrhagic ovarian cyst.
Ruptured ovarian cyst.
Acute pelvic inflammatory disease

b. Serum β-HCG.
Ultrasound scan.
Microbiology swabs – endocervical, high vaginal and urethral.
Diagnostic laparoscopy.

c. Ectopic gestation: surgery/conservative medical treatment.
Acute pelvic inflammatory disease: antibiotics (covering Gram-negative

and -positive bacteria, *Chlamydia*
and *Bacteroides*).

Ovarian cyst: ovarian cystectomy or
oophorectomy.

Question 9

a. Aria-Stella phenomenon.
b. Ectopic gestation.
   Progestogen treatment.
c. Reassess her symptoms.
   Measure β-HCG.
d. Diagnostic laparoscopy.

Question 10

a. Recurrent miscarriage.
b. Uterine hypoplasia.
c. Ultrasound of the pelvic organs.
   Ultrasound of the kidneys and ureters.
   Intravenous urogram.
   Hysteroscopy.
d. None.
e. She is likely to have miscarriages until
   she is able to carry a pregnancy beyond
   viability.

Infertility and gynaecological endocrinology

Question 1

a. Hysterosalpingogram.
b. Bilateral hydrosalpinges.
c. *Chlamydia trachomatis.*
   Neisseria gonorrhoeae.
d. Appendicitis.
   Postabortal pelvic infection.
   Postpartum infection.
   After the insertion of an intrauterine
      contraceptive device.
e. *In vitro* fertilization and embryo
   transfer (IVF-ET).
f. Adoption.

Question 2

a. Intracytoplasmic sperm
   injection/microassisted fertilization.
b. Severe oligospermia.
   Azoospermia (sperm only being

available in minute numbers having
been aspirated from the testicle or
epididymis).

Repeated failure to fertilize at IVF when
sperms and eggs seem to be 'normal'.
c. Adoption.
   Donor insemination.
   Embryo donation.
   Stop treatment.
d. Up to 30%.

Question 3

a. Gamete intrafallopian transfer.
b. The fallopian tube(s) must be patent
   and appear normal.
c. Written consent of the providers of the
   eggs and sperm.
d. Used by the surviving partner.
   Be allowed to perish.
   Donated for use by others.
   Used for licensed research.

Question 4

a. Polycystic ovarian syndrome.
b. Obesity.
   Hirsutism.
   Acne.
   Baldness.
c. Ultrasound scan of the ovaries.
   Hormone profile (luteinizing hormone
      (LH), follicle-stimulating hormone
      (FSH), testosterone,
      androstenedione, serum-hormone-
      binding globulin).
d. Anovulation.
e. Clomiphene citrate.
   FSH alone or with down-regulation
      with LHRH analogues.
   Surgery (wedge resection or
      electrodiathermy or laser of the
      ovaries).
   Weight loss.

Question 5

a. Polycystic ovarian syndrome.
b. Hirsutism.
   Male-type baldness.
   Acne.

c. Mechanical methods – shaving/
    electrolysis/waxing.
    Spironolactone.
    Reverse sequential therapy
    (cyproterone acetate and oestrogens).
d. Diabetes mellitus.
    Endometrial carcinoma.
    Ischaemic heart disease.
e. Combined oral contraceptive pill
f. Maintain correct weight.
    She may have difficulties in conceiving
    and therefore may require ovulation
    induction.
    She will require regular medical check-
    ups to enable early identification of
    diabetes mellitus or endometrial
    carcinoma.

Question 6

a. Amenorrhoea of at least six months
    following regular cycles.
b. Hyperprolactinaemia.
c. MRI of the pituitary fossa.
    CT scan if claustrophobic.
d. Bromocriptine.
    Cabergoline.
    Quinagolide.
e. Start bromocriptine with 1.0–1.25 mg
    at bedtime and gradually increase the
    dose to a maximum of 30 mg/day (as
    divided doses).
    Start cabergoline at 500 µg weekly as a
    single dose or two divided doses and
    increase to a maximum of 4.5 mg (as
    divided doses).
    Start quinagolide at 25 µg at bedtime
    and increase at intervals of three days
    in steps of 25 µg to a maintenance
    dose of 75–150 µg daily
    (occasionally maximum dose may be
    up to 300 µg).
f. Drugs, e.g phenothiazines.
    Steroids (e.g. contraceptive pills,
    Depo-Provera).
    Pituitary adenomas (prolactinomas).
    Hypothyroidism.
    Craniopharyngioma
    Stress.
    Fracture of the base of the skull.

Question 7

a. Oligospermia.
    Teratozoospermia (high proportion of
    abnormal sperms – normal sperms
    should be at least 30%).
    Asthenozoospermia (poor motility –
    normal sperms should be at least
    40%).
b. Repeat the semen analysis, preferably
    after three days of abstinence, and also
    ensure that the sample is delivered to
    the lab within one hour of collection.
c. Take a history from the man looking
    specifically for factors such as
    alcohol intake, smoking, long hot
    baths, long distance driving on a
    heated seat and stress, and then do a
    physical examination.
    Investigate the female partner to
    confirm that she is ovulating.
d. Attempt to improve motility by
    removing day factors identified from
    history.
    Treat with vitamin C 250 mg daily or
    vitamin E 800 mg daily to remove
    free radicals.
    IVF (if tubes are not patent) but couple
    must be prepared for failure of
    fertilization.
    Intracytoplasmic sperm injection (this
    may be the most successful treatment
    for the couple).
e. Serum FSH/LH, testosterone.
    Testicular biopsy.
    Karyotype.
    Vasogram.

Question 8

a. Azoospermia.
b. Gonadal dysgenesis.
    Obstruction of the seminiferous tubules
    (e.g. by infection).
    Post-vasectomy.
    Seminiferous tubule failure.
    Post-surgery (orchidectomy, other
    groin surgery).
    Congenital absence of the vas deferens
    Drugs, e.g. chemotherapy.
    Radiotherapy.

c. FSH/LH, testosterone.
    Testicular biopsy.
    Karyotype.
d. Intracytoplasmic sperm injection if the
    problem is due to obstruction.
    Donor insemination.
    Embryo donation.
    Adoption.
    Stop all treatment.

Question 9

a. Anovulation.
b. Cervical mucus – spinnbarkeit.
    Serial pelvic ultrasound tracking to
    demonstrate failure of follicle
    development.
    Luteal phase endometrial biopsy.
c. Polycystic ovarian syndrome.
    Hyperprolactinaemia.
    Hypothyroidism.
    Drugs (e.g. after taking the pill or other
    contraceptives).
    Pituitary adenomas (prolactinomas).
    Weight loss.
    Ovarian failure.
d. Clomiphene citrate.
    Gonadotrophins with or without
    down-regulation.
e. Multiple pregnancies.
    Possible increased incidence of ovarian
    carcinoma with prolonged treatment
    with clomiphene citrate.
    Ovarian hyperstimulation syndrome.

Question 10

a. Tubal patency test.
b. Hysterosalpingography.
    HyCoSy using echovist or saline.
    Diagnostic laparoscopy and dye
    test.
c. Hysterosalpingography: outpatient
    procedure requiring no general
    anaesthesia which outlines uterine
    cavity and tubes. Employs contrast
    and X-ray. May demonstrate uterine
    synechiae. Does not demonstrate
    pelvic adhesions reliably or pelvic
    pathology. High incidence of false
    positives because of tubal spasm.

Patient may suffer from vasovagal
attack.
HyCoSy: demonstrates uterine cavity
and tubes, and also screens for
ovarian or uterine abnormalities such
as cysts and fibroids, respectively.
Employs ultrasound and either
echovist or saline. Does not
demonstrate pelvic adhesions.
Laparoscopy and dye test:
demonstrates extrinsic tubal and
other pelvic pathology such as
adhesions, endometriosis and
subserous fibroids. Involves
anaesthesia (general anaesthesia in
most centres) and does not screen for
intrauterine and intrinsic tubal
pathology.
d. Post-coital test.
    Endometrial biopsy in the luteal phase.
    Hormone profile in the proliferative
    phase.

Endometriosis

Question 1

a. Endometriosis.
b. Secondary dysmenorrhoea.
    Menstrual abnormality.
    Deep dyspareunia.
c. Infertility.
d. Continuous progestogens.
    Continuous combined oral
    contraceptive pill.
    Danazol.
    LHRH analogues.
    Laser/diathermy to the endometriotic
    tissue.
e. Sampson's implantation theory.
    Coelomic metaplastic theory.
    Vascular/lymphatic theory.

Question 2

a. Duration, site, character of pain and
    relationship with periods; regularity of
    cycles, infertility and deep dyspareunia.
b. Bluish spots on the vagina or cervix.
    Fixed retroverted uterus.

Cervical excitation tenderness.
Bulky uterus.
Tenderness in both adnexa.
Indurated nodules in utero-sacral
    ligaments.
c. Diagnostic laparoscopy.
d. Endometriosis externa.
    Adenomyosis.
    Pelvic inflammatory disease.
    Submucous fibroids.

Question 3

a. It occurs in about 15% of women with
    infertility.
b. There is an association between
    infertility and endometriosis.
c. Continuous progestogens.
    Continuous combined oral
        contraceptive pill.
    LHRH analogues.
d. Headaches.
    Acne.
    Muscle cramps.
    Reduction in breast size.
    Voice changes (this may, however, be
        permanent).
    Hirsutism
e. She must avoid pregnancy as danazol
    could androgenize a female fetus.

Pelvic inflammatory disease and genitourinary medicine

Question 1

a. Vulval warts.
b. Lumps on the vulva.
    Pruritus vulvulae.
    Superficial dyspareunia.
c. Human papilloma virus.
d. Vagina, cervix, anal region and the
    mouth.
e. Cervical smear.
f. Carcinoma of the vulva.

Question 2

a. Acute pelvic inflammatory disease.
b. *Chlamydia* infection.

Neisseria gonorrhoeae.
c. Endocervical swab.
    High vaginal swab.
    Urethral/rectal swab.
    Serum for *Chlamydia* antibodies.
    Veneral Disease Research Laboratory
        (VDRL) serology.
d. She is likely to have Fitz–Hugh–Curtis
    syndrome (perihepatitis).
e. Doxycycline.
    Ciprofloxacin (Ciproxin) –
        4-quinolone derivatives.
    Erythromycin.
    Azithromycin.

Question 3

a. Lower abdominal pain.
    Vaginal discharge.
    Deep dyspareunia.
    Dysmenorrhoea.
    Menorrhagia.
    Infertility.
b. *Chlamydia trachomatis.*
    Neisseria gonorrhoeae.
c. Antibiotics to cover both organisms.
d. Bilateral hydrosalpinges from chronic
    pelvic inflammatory disease.

Question 4

a. Intracellular Gram-positive diplococci
    (*Neisseria gonorrhoeae*).
b. Vaginal discharge.
    Asymptomatic (sexual partner
        symptomatic).
    Generalized malaise/pyrexia.
    Abdominal pain.
c. Doxycycline.
    Cefuroxime.
    Ciprofloxacin (Ciproxin).
d. Contact tracing.
    Screen for other sexually transmitted
        diseases.

Question 5

a. *Trichomonas vaginalis.*
b. Vaginal discharge which may be
        malodorous.
    Soreness of the vulva.

Vulvovaginal pruritis.

Superficial dyspareunia.

c. Erythematous vulva.

Greenish-yellow foul-smelling discharge.

Punctate haemorrhages on the cervix/vagina.

d. Metronidazole 400 mg tds for seven days.

e. She may experience nausea, a metallic or a disagreeable taste.

She must avoid alcohol.

If she must have sexual intercourse, a condom must be used.

Her partner needs to be treated.

Question 6

a. Counselling about HIV infection.

b. Multiple sexual partners.

Intravenous drug abuser.

Sexual contact with someone from Africa within the last 12 months.

Bisexuals and haemophiliacs.

c. One to five years.

d. Opportunistic infections (bacteria, fungi, parasites and viruses).

Kaposi's sarcoma.

e. Retrovirus (human T-cell lymphotrophic virus).

Question 7

a. Lymphadenopathy.

Ulcers on the cervix.

b. Syphilis

c. Swab from the ulcers for dark field microscopy.

Serology – VDRL.

Fluorescent treponemal antibody absorption test (FTA-ABS).

d. Parenteral penicillin.

e. Secondary syphilis.

Tertiary syphilis: cardiovascular, neurological and other systemic manifestations.

Question 8

a. *Neisseria gonorrhoeae.*

b. None.

Vaginal discharge.

Dysuria.

Abdominal pain.

Malaise.

Fever.

c. Urethral swab.

Rectal swab.

High vaginal swab.

d. *Chlamydia trachomatis.*

Trichomonas vaginalis.

HIV.

Other sexually transmitted diseases.

e. Antibiotics (cefuroxime/ciprofl oxacin).

Contact tracing.

Question 9

a. Younger age at initiation of sexual intercourse.

Greater number of sexual partners.

Failure to use barrier contraceptives.

Higher prevalence of *Neisseria gonorrhoeae* and *Chlamydia trachomatis.*

Smoking.

Alcohol and drugs.

b. Combined oral contraceptive pill.

Condoms and other barrier methods of contraception.

c. *Chlamydia trachomatis.*

Neisseria gonorrhoeae.

Mycoplasma hominis.

Ureaplasma urealyticum.

Mycobacterium tuberculosis.

d. Chronic pelvic pain.

Deep dyspareunia.

Heavy and irregular/painful periods.

Ectopic pregnancy.

Infertility.

Question 10

a. *Mycobacterium tuberculosis.*

b. Chest pain.

Chronic cough.

Weight loss.

Night sweats.

Asymptomatic.

c. Chest X-ray.

Endometrial biopsy for Ziehl–Nielsen stain and histology (looking for tubercles).
Mantoux test.
d. The chest, with haematogenous spread to the pelvis.
e. Rifampicin, isoniazid and pyrazinamide.
f. Very poor.

Genital prolapse and urinary incontinence

Question 1
a. Physical examination to exclude prolapse.
Urine microscopy.
Urodynamic investigation.
b. Genuine stress incontinence.
c. Normal bladder capacity.
Normal initial sensation to void.
No leakage during filling.
Leakage of urine when asked to raised intra-abdominal pressure.
d. Weight loss (if she is obese).
Pelvic floor exercises.
Surgery (colposuspension or Stamey's operation).

Question 2
a. Detrusor instability.
b. Urinary tract infection.
Genuine stress incontinence.
Low compliance bladder.
c. Urine microscopy, culture and sensitivity (MCS).
Blood glucose.
Uridynamics.
d. Bladder drill.
Anticholinergics.
Calcium channel blockers.
Tricyclic antidepressants.
Oestrogen cream/HRT.

Question 3
a. Uterine descent with cervix outside the introitus but the body still within the vagina.

b. Lump in the vagina.
Dragging sensation in the vagina.
Backache.
Urinary frequency and nocturia.
Bloody vaginal discharge.
c. Abdominal masses/ascites.
Urethrocele.
Decubitus ulcer.
Cystocele.
Enterocele.
Rectocele.
d. Support with a vaginal pessary.
Surgery – vaginal hysterectomy and repair or Manchester repair.

Question 4
a. Detrusor instability.
b. Mid-stream urine specimen (MSU) for MCS.
Blood glucose.
c. Frequency.
Nocturia.
Urgency and urge incontinence.
Stress incontinence.
d. Oxybutynin hydrochloride or Pro-Banthine.
e. Blurred vision.
Constipation.

Question 5
a. Vesicovaginal fistula.
b. Intravenous urogram.
Dye test under general anaesthesia.
c. Intravenous urogram or ultrasound scan of the kidneys.
MSU to exclude infection.
d. Bladder calculi.
Recurrent urinary tract infections.
Severe psychosocial problems.
Atrophic bladder.

Question 6
a. Genital prolapse.
b. Decubitus ulcer.
c. Ulceration after dependent oedema.
d. Ensure that the ulcer is not infected.
e. Oestrogen deficiency.
Childbirth.

Obesity.
Chronic cough.
Abdominal masses and ascites.

Question 7

a. Vaginal ulceration.
   Retention of urine.
b. Retention of urine.
   Difficulties with removing pessary
     (retention).
   Vaginal ulceration.
c. Where the patient is unsuitable for
     surgery.
   To allow decubitus ulceration to heal
     before surgery.
   In pregnancy.
   To alleviate symptoms while awaiting
     surgery.
d. It should be changed at least every 3–6
   months. This is mainly to ensure that
   there are no ulcers and that the
   pessaries are not forgotten. Usually,
   with time, smaller pessaries may need
   to be inserted otherwise they become
   very difficult to replace.

Question 8

a. Low compliance bladder/detrusor
   instability.
b. Anticholinergic drugs, e.g. Ditropan
   (oxybutynin hydrochloride).
   Intermittent self-catheterization (if
     large residual urine).
   Complex cystocaecoplasty.
   Urinary diversion.
   Sacral nerve cystoplasty.
c. Multiple sclerosis.
d. Cystoscopy.
   Pelvic nerve assessment.

Family planning and psychosexual medicine

Question 1

a. When did you have sexual intercourse?
   When was the first day of your last
     menstrual period?

b. PC4.
   Combined oral contraceptive pill.
   Intrauterine contraceptive device.
c. To take two now and another two after
     12 hours.
   If there is any vomiting, she must take
     two more tablets.
   If she fails to menstruate at the expected
     time, she must report to a doctor.
d. They may reduce absorption from the
     bowel by eliminating gut flora.
   They may affect liver metabolism.
e. Provide her with a definitive method of
     contraception or arrange an
     appointment for her at the local family
     planning clinic or with her GP.

Question 2

a. Intrauterine contraceptive device
     (multiload copper IUCD).
b. Unexplained uterine bleeding.
   Pregnancy.
   Pelvic inflammatory disease.
   Previous ectopic pregnancy.
   Enlarged uterus (e.g. due to fibroids).
   Allergy to copper.
c. Irregular vaginal bleeding.
   Intermenstrual bleeding.
   Expulsion.
   Perforation of the uterus.
   Pelvic inflammatory disease.
d. To feel the thread after every period.

Question 3

a. She could be pregnant.
   The device has been expelled.
   The device and its thread have migrated
     up into the uterine cavity.
   The device has migrated into the
     peritoneal cavity through a
     perforation.
b. Feeling the cavity of the uterus with a
     sound.
   Ultrasound.
   Hysterosalpingogram using another
     intrauterine contraceptive device or a
     uterine sound as a marker.
   Hysteroscopy.

Plane abdominal X-ray using a uterine sound or an intrauterine contraceptive device as a marker.
c. If the device is inert, leave alone provided the patient is asymptomatic.
    If it is a copper device, it has to be removed.
d. During insertion (especially after a termination or soon after delivery) and most likely by the push-through method of insertion rather than the pull-out method.

Question 4
a. Take out the device if the thread is visible.
    Allow the pregnancy to progress with the device *in situ*.
b. If the device is removed, she may miscarry.
    If the device is left *in situ*, she may miscarry and be at a higher risk of antepartum haemorrhage or premature rupture of membranes.

Question 5
a, Norplant.
b. Five years.
c. Levonorgestrel.
d. Irregular vaginal bleeding.
    Amenorrhoea.
    Weight gain.
    Acne.
e. Pregnancy.
    Irregular periods.
    Unexplained uterine bleeding.
    Active liver disease.
f. A failure rate of 0.03 per hundred woman years.

Question 6
a. One in 300.
b. Laparoscopy.
    Minilaparotomy.
    Posterior colpotomy.
c. Falope rings.
    Filshie clips.
    Hulka Clemens clips.

d. Increased risk of ectopic pregnancy if the procedure fails.
    If the woman has been taking the pill, her periods may be heavier.
    Complications of laparoscopy (trauma to blood vessels, bladder, bowel; gas embolism, subcutaneous emphysema, etc.).
e. The type of anaesthesia used.
    Vasectomy is an alternative which the couple should consider.
    After the procedure, she is unlikely to be accepted for reversal.

Question 7
a. Cervical cap: genital prolapse, allergy to the device. Failure rate: 3–12 per 100 woman years.
b. Progestogen-only pill: unexplained vaginal bleeding, past or current severe arterial disease, pregnancy – actual or possible. Failure rate: 2–4 per 100 woman years.
c. Progestogen-only intrauterine contraceptive device (Mirena): unexplained vaginal bleeding, pregnancy (actual or possible), enlarged uterus. Failure rate: 0.14 per 100 woman years.
d. Combined oral contraceptive pill: previous deep venous thrombosis, pregnancy (actual or possible), oestrogen-dependent tumour, chronic or active liver disease, past or current severe arterial disease, undiagnosed genital tract bleeding. Failure rate: 0.1–0.4 per 100 women years.
e. Diaphragm: prolapse, unexplained vaginal bleeding, prolapse, allergy to device. Failure rate: 3–12 per 100 woman years.

Question 8
a. Hypoactive sexual desire.
    Arousal disorder.
    Sexual aversion disorder.
    Inhibited orgasm.
    Vaginismus.
    Dyspareunia.

b. Erectile dysfunction.
 Premature ejaculation.
 Inhibited orgasm or retarded
   ejaculation.
 Hypoactive sexual desire.
c. Physical causes.
 Relationship factors.
 Ignorance.
 Negative attitudes.
 Psychological factors.
 Psychiatric disturbances.
d. Psychotherapy.
 Intracavernousal injection therapy with
   prostaglandins, etc.
 Vacuum tumescence therapy.
 Penile implants.
 Hormone treatment (if
   hypoandrogenic).

Menopause

Question 1
a. Premature menopause.
b. Hot flushes.
 Dryness of the vagina.
 Superficial dyspareunia.
 Urinary symptoms (frequency and
   urgency).
 Irritability.
 Fatigue.
 Insomnia.
 Mood swings.
 Memory loss.
c. HRT with oestrogens and
   progestogens.
d. Alleviation of vasomotor symptoms.
 Prevention of genital atrophy.
 Protection against cardiovascular
   disease.
 Prevention of osteoporosis.
 Protection against Alzhiemer's disease.

Question 2
a. Osteoporosis.
 Cardiovascular disease.
 Vasomotor symptoms (hot flushes,
   night sweats, irritability, memory
   loss).

 Genital atrophy.
 Dry vagina and dyspareunia.
 Dry skin and loss of hair.
 Alzhiemer's disease.
b. Tablets.
 Transdermal patches.
 Implants.
c. Active breast cancer.
 Acute phase deep venous thrombosis.
 Acute phase pulmonary embolus.
 Active liver disease.
 Undiagnosed breast lump.
 Undiagnosed vaginal bleeding.
d. For a minimum of 10 years.

Question 3
a. Ovestin (oestrogen).
b. Atrophic vaginitis.
 Atrophic cervicitis.
 Preparation of the vagina for surgery
   for prolapse.
 Insertion of pessaries.
 Urinary incontinence.
c. Endometrial hyperplasia.
 Endometrial carcinoma.
d. Active breast cancer.
 Severe active liver disease.
 Undiagnosed vaginal bleeding.
 Undiagnosed breast lump.
 Active endometrial cancer.

Question 4
a. Atrophic vaginitis and ectocervicitis.
 HRT.
b. Pipelle endometrial biopsy.
 Hysteroscopy and endometrial biopsy.
 Ultrasound scan.
c. Oral progestogen therapy.
 Progestogen-only intrauterine
   contraceptive device (Mirena).
d. Atypical endometrial hyperplasia.
 Endometrial carcinoma.
 Ovarian carcinoma.
 Carcinoma of the cervix.

Question 5
a. Early age at menopause.
 Family history.
 Smoking.

Lack of exercise.

Small stature.

Hysterectomy with or without bilateral salpingo-ophorectomy.

b. Bone densitometry.

c. Exercise.

Adequate dietary intake of calcium.

HRT after menopause.

d. Testosterone implants.

Livial.

e. The risk of developing deep venous thrombosis is three times greater in women on HRT than in non-menstruating age-matched controls, but is less than that during the reproductive age.

The risk of breast cancer is only slightly higher after 10 years of HRT.

Question 6

a. No.

b. Endometrial hyperplasia.

Irregular vaginal bleeding.

Breast tenderness.

Deep venous thrombosis.

Weight gain.

c. By the addition of progestogens to the treatment.

d. By regular breast examination.

By ensuring that any new symptoms are reported promptly and investigated.

Gynaecological tumours (benign and malignant)

Question 1

a. Reassure her that she does not have cancer.

The abnormality is mild and may spontaneously revert to normal.

The smear should be repeated in six months.

If a second smear suggests an abnormality, she would be referred for colposcopy, directed biopsy, treatment and follow-up.

b. Moderate dykaryosis.

Severe dyskaryosis.

Smear report with suggestion of invasive disease.

c. May have a blood-stained discharge for up to two weeks.

Avoid sexual intercourse for two weeks.

Not to use tampons with next period.

She requires close follow-up with repeat smears.

Reassure her that there will be no long-term effects on her fertility or future pregnancies.

Question 2

a. When the whole of the transformation zone cannot be identified on colposcopy.

When an endocervical lesion extends up the canal.

When invasion or microinvasion cannot be excluded.

When a colposcope is unavailable.

b. Haemorrhage.

Infection.

Cervical stenosis.

Cervical incompetence.

Subfertility or infertility.

c. Cone biopsies are performed under general anaesthesia.

LLETZ is unlikely to be associated with fertility or cervical complications.

d. Cryocautery.

Diathermy.

Laser.

Cold (Semm) coagulation.

Question 3

a. Invasive carcinoma of the cervix.

b. Biopsy and histology.

c Examination under anaesthesia.

Cystoscopy.

Rectal examination.

d. Ultrasound scan of the kidneys and liver.

CT scan.

Intravenous urogram.

Chest X-ray.
Urea and electrolytes.
e. Wertheim's hysterectomy.
Radiotherapy.

Question 4

a. Pipelle endometrial biopsy (it must be
recognized that because of the
fibrotic nature of the lesions, this
sampling method tends to be
inadequate).
Ultrasound scan of the pelvic organs.
Hysteroscopy and endometrial biopsy.
b. Endometrial polyp.
Endometrial hyperplasia.
Endometrial carcinoma.
Adenomyosis.
Endometrial sarcoma.
c. Hysterectomy for atypical hyperplasia
or malignancy.
For benign conditions, endometrial
curettage and polpectomy.

Question 5

a. The risk to any woman developing
ovarian cancer by the age of 70 is one in
120, increasing to one in 40 with one
first degree relative affected. Miss K has
two first degree relatives affected and
this increases her lifetime risk to
approximately 40%.
b. Use of the combined oral contraceptive
pill.
Avoidance of ovulation induction drugs
such as clomiphene citrate.
Bearing children.
c. There is no satisfactory screening
method available. However, the
currently available methods include:
serum CA125;
ultrasound scan and Doppler
ultrasound of the ovaries;
pelvic examination in the
post-menopausal woman;
genetic screening for BRCA1 and
BRCA2 where family members have
been affected.
d. Bilateral salpingo-ophorectomy (with

hysterectomy) after she has completed
her family.

Question 6

a. Hydatidiform mole.
b. Full blood count.
Blood group and cross match.
Liver function test.
Coagulation profile.
Baseline blood and urine β-HCG.
Chest X-ray.
c. Suction evacuation of the uterus.
d. Registration with a trophoblastic centre
(Sheffield, Dundee or Charing Cross,
London).
Serial urinary β-HCG estimations.
Avoidance of pregnancy for at least 6
months.

Question 7

a. Ovarian carcinoma.
b. Loss of appetite.
Pelvic pain.
Weight loss.
Dyspepsia.
Pressure symptoms.
Urinary frequency.
Constipation.
Hormone effects (abnormal vaginal
bleeding or virilization).
c. Chest X-ray.
Serum CA125.
Liver function tests.
Renal function tests.
CT scan.
d. Growth involves one or both ovaries
and there is intraperitoneal spread
outside the pelvis. Histologically this
can also be confirmed by the presence
of tumour on the small bowel or
omentum if tumour is confined to the
true pelvis.

Question 8

a. At least stage IIIb.
b. Palliative surgery.
Intracavitary and external radiation.
c. Diarrhoea/rectal bleeding/tenesmus.

Symptoms of cystitis – frequency,
urgency, haematuria, dysuria.
Malaise/loss of appetite.
Flare-up of pelvic inflammatory
disease.
d. Proctocolitis.
Subacute bowel obstruction/small
bowel perforation.
Cystitis.
Fistula (vesicovaginal or rectovaginal).
Loss of ovarian function.
Gynaetresia (narrowing of the vagina)
leading to either dyspareunia or
apareunia.

Question 9
a. Obesity.
Diabetes mellitus.
Nulliparity.
Exogenous unopposed oestrogens.
Anovulatory disorders including
polycystic ovarian syndrome.
Early menarche.
Late menopause.
Hypertension.
b. Total abdominal hysterectomy and
bilateral salpingo-ophorectomy.
(Peritoneal cytology, omentotomy,
lymphatic node sampling if
indicated).
c. Radiotherapy.
d. FIGO stage Ic.
e. Poor differentiation.
Invasion into the outer half of the
myometrium.

Question 10
a. Obvious invasive cancer involving the
cervix only.
b. Removal of the uterus, cervix, upper
vagina, parametrium and lymph nodes.
Ovaries are likely to be conserved (in
view of her age).
c. Complications of anaesthesia.
Haemorrhage.
Injury to the ureter(s) and bladder.
Peritonitis.
Ileus.

Intestinal obstruction.
Thromboembolism.
Urinary tract infection.
d. Vesicovaginal fistula.
Ureteric stenosis.
Lymphocyst formation.
Lymphoedema.
Ovarian remnant syndrome.
e. If the lymph nodes are free, this will not
be required. If they are involved, then
radiotherapy will be required.
In the absence of node involvement, the
five-year survival is 80%. Where the
nodes are involved, the five-year
survival is 50%.

Question 11
a. Torsion of an ovarian (dermoid) cyst.
b. Dermoid cyst.
Fibroids.
Tubo-ovarian mass (pyosalpinx or
hydrosalpinx).
Mesenteric cysts.
Appendix abscess.
Broad ligament tumour.
Endometriosis cysts.
Haemorrhagic corpus luteum cyst.
Pelvic kidney.
c. Plain X-ray of the abdomen which may
demonstrate a tooth.
d. Confirmation of diagnosis by
laparoscopy.
Laparotomy and cystectomy if the
ovary is still viable or oophorectomy
if it is not. Cystectomy can also be
performed laparoscopically.
e. Germ cell tumours which are
commonly benign but malignant forms
do occasionally arise. They are the most
common tumour of the ovary in the
reproductive age group.

Question 12
a. Pipelle endometrial biospy.
Ultrasound scan.
Hysteroscopy and endometrial biospy.
b. Hysterectomy and bilateral salpingo-
ophorectomy.

c. Radiation in a patient who is unfit for
   surgery.
   Provera in an extremely unfit patient.
d. Grade 3 histology.
   Deep myometrial invasion.
   Lymph node metastases.
   Spread beyond the uterus.
   Histological clear cell type.

Question 13
a. Full blood count.
   Liver function tests.
   CA125.
   Urea and electrolytes.
   Ultrasound scan.
   Ascitic tap for cytology.
b. Surgery involves a vertical incision.
   Uterus, tubes, ovaries and omentum
      should be removed.
   Bowel resection may be necessary.
   Overall aim is to debulk tumour as
      much as possible.
c. Chemotherapy consisting of platinum
   compounds either as single agents or in
   combination with other antimitotic
   agents.
d. The five-year survival rate is less than
   5%.

Question 14
a. Multiple uterine fibroids.
b. Ultrasound scan.
c. None.
   Pressure symptoms (urinary frequency,
      constipation).
   Intermenstrual bleeding (only if
      submucous).
   Abdominal pain (only if degeneration
      or submucous).
   Symptoms of anaemia or
      polycythaemia.
d. Myomectomy.
e. Haemorrhage which may progress to
   hysterectomy.
f. By offering her preoperative LHRH
   analogues for 3–6 months to reduce
   the size and vascularity of the
   fibroids.

Question 15
a. Cervical fibroid polyp.
b. Lower abdominal dragging pain.
   Lump in the vagina.
   Intermenstrual bleeding.
   Heavy periods.
   Vaginal discharge.
c. Torsion.
   Ulceration.
   Infection.
   Calcification.
   Sarcomatous degeneration.
d. Removal of the polyp.

Question 16
a. Ovarian fibroma.
b. Meigs' syndrome.
c. Pelvic ultrasound scan.
d. Ascites.
   Pyrexia.
e. Removal of the fibroma. This is usually
   followed by the disappearance of the
   ascites, hydrothorax and pyrexia.

Question 17
a. Atypical endometrial hyperplasia.
b. Unopposed oestrogen therapy.
   Oestrogen-producing tumours.
   Anovulatory conditions.
c. There is a 15–40% risk of progression
   to malignancy.
d. Hysterectomy and bilateral
   salpingo-ophorectomy.
e. Diabetes mellitus.
   Polycystic ovarian disease.
   Tamoxifen therapy.
   Unopposed oestrogen therapy for
   HRT.

Question 18
a. Masculinization.
b. Adrenal tumours.
   Masculinizing tumours of the ovary.
c. Ultrasound scan of the ovaries and
   adrenals.
   CT scan of the ovaries and adrenals.
   Serum androstenedione.
d. Hirsutism.

Muscle cramps.
Male-type baldness.
Brittle hair.
e. Removal of the ovarian or adrenal
   tumour.

Question 19
a. Carcinoma of the cervix.
b. Endometrial carcinoma.
c. Carcinoma of the vulvar.
d. Simple hyperplasia.
e. Choriocarcinoma.

Question 20
a. An endodermal sinus tumour (germ cell
   tumour).
b. Dysgerminoma.
   Immature teratoma.
   Matured cystic teratoma with
      malignant transformation.
   Embryonal carcinoma.
   Choriocarcinoma.
c. Unilateral salpingo-ophorectomy
   followed by chemotherapy.
d. Serial serum alpha-fetoprotein
      measurements.
   Regular clinical and radiological
      assessments.

Vulvar disorders

Question 1
a. Vulvar carcinoma.
b. Squamous cell carcinoma.
   Adenocarcinoma.
   Melanoma.
c. Human papilloma virus infection.
   Vulvar intraepithelial neoplasia.
   Non-neoplastic vulval diseases such as
      squamous hyperplasia and lichen
      sclerosus et atrophicus with atypia.
d. Surgery – most commonly radical
      vulvar excision with groin dissection.
   Adjuvant radiotherapy will be offered if
      there are more than one positive
      groin lymph nodes.

e. The five-year survival is over 90% in
   the absence of groin node involvement.

Question 2
a. Burning sensation in the vulva.
   Discomfort.
   White patch on the vulva.
   Superficial dyspareunia.
b. It belongs to the non-neoplastic
   epithelial disorders of the vulva. These
   include lichen sclerosus, squamous cell
   hyperplasia and other dermatoses.
c. White, crinkly plaques.
   Shrinkage of vulval structures.
   Thinned vulval skin.
d. Topical corticosteroid cream.
   Topical oestrogen creams.
   Topical testosterone cream.
e. The role of surgery is very limited.
f. Treatment is difficult but progression to
   malignancy is said to occur in less than
   5%.

Question 3
a. Vulval pain.
   Soreness.
   Discomfort.
   Asymptomatic.
b. Vulvar intraepithelial neoplasia.
   Non-neoplastic epithelial disorders.
c. Cervical cytology.
   Colposcopic assessment of the genital
      tract (vagina and cervix).
   Vulvoscopy and biopsy to exclude
      invasive disease.
d. Small asymptomatic lesions should be
      managed by observation alone.
   Topical steroids, lignocaine gel or
      amitriptyline for small asymptomatic
      lesions.
   Laser vaporization.
   Excisional therapy.
e. Regular vulvoscopy and biopsy of
      abnormal areas.
   Regular cervical cytology and
      colposcopy.
   The rate of progression to invasive

disease is estimated to be as high as 10% in cases of VIN3 and may occur more than five years after the initial diagnosis. Long-term follow-up is therefore recommended.

Question 4

a. Bartholin's abscess.
b. *Neisseria gonorrhoeae.*
   Escherichia coli.
   Staphylococcus aureus.
   Streptoccocus faecalis.
   Trichomonas vaginalis.
c. Local discomfort.
   Acutely tender swelling.
   Superficial dyspareunia.
   Vaginal discharge.
d. Antibiotics.
   Marsupialization.

Question 5

a. *Candida albicans.*
b. Soreness of the vagina/vulva.
   Thick white cheesy vaginal discharge.
   Vulval pruritus.
   Superficial dyspareunia.
c. Thick white plaques on the vaginal wall.
   Haemorrhagic spots on the vagina.
   Oedema or diffusely reddened vagina.
d. Use of combined oral contraceptive pill.
   Use of broad-spectrum antibiotics.
   Pregnancy.
   Immunosuppressive therapy.
   Diabetes mellitus.
e. Clotrimazole.
   Nystatin.
   Ketoconazole.

Question 6

a. Cervical polyp.
   Fibroid polyp.
   Vulval lipoma.
   Vaginal polyp.
b. Decubitus ulcer.
c. Examination under anaesthesia.
d. Excision of the polyp.

Hysterectomy.
Packing to encourage healing of the ulcer and antibiotics.
Replacement of the prolapse with a pessary.

Gynaecological surgery

Question 1

a. Low haemoglobin.
   High platelet count.
   Microcytic hypochromic red blood cells.
b. Pelvic examination.
   Coagulation profile.
   Serum ferritin.
c. Combined oral contraceptive pill.
   Tranexamic acid 1 g four times a day during menstruation.
   Ferrous sulphate or ferrous gluconate.
d. Danazol 200–400 mg twice daily.
   LHRH analogues.
e. Adenomyosis.

Question 2

a. Cough, chest pain and shortness of breath.
   Dysuria, frequency, nocturia and haematuria.
   Painful and/or discharging wound.
   Abdominal swelling or pelvic pain.
   Leg pain or swelling.
b. Respiratory infection.
   Wound infection.
   Infected pelvic haematoma.
   Urinary tract infection.
   Deep venous thrombosis.
c. Full blood count.
   Blood culture.
   Urine for microscopy and culture.
   Chest X-ray if there are chest symptoms.
   Sputum culture.
   Ultrasound to exclude an infected haematoma.
   Wound swabs.

Doppler of the relevant vessels if there is a suspicion of deep venous thrombosis.

d. Antibiotics and conservative management.

Question 3

a. Bilateral loin pains radiating to the suprapubic region.
  Vaginal bleeding.
  Severe generalized abdominal pain.
  Suprapubic pain.
b. Sweaty/cold extremities/pallor.
  Tachycardia.
  Hypotension.
  Tenderness over the kidney area.
  Abdominal distension.
  Generalized abdominal tenderness.
  Dullness to percussion in the suprapubic area.
c. Bilateral ligation of the ureters.
  Severe intra-abdominal haemorrhage complicated by acute renal failure.
  Catheter blockage.
d. Ureteric ligation: intravenous urogram.
  Haemorrhage: resuscitate with intravenous fluids and crossmatch blood (at least 4 units). Arrange an exploratory laparotomy.
  Catheter blockage: flush/change catheter.

Question 4

a. Rollen's spatula: cervical smear.
b. Pipelle: endometrial biopsy.
c. Ring pessary: support of a prolapsed uterus.
d. Sims' speculum: exposure of the vaginal walls and cervix.
e. Uterine sound: used to determine the size and axis of the uterus.
f. Shelf pessary: to support a prolapsed uterus.
g. Cusco's bivalve speculum: used to expose the cervix and vaginal walls.
h. Uterine currette: for biopsy of the endometrium.
i. Trocar and cannular: for insertion of oestrogen implants.
j. Cytobrush: for cervical smear where the cervix is stenosed or the squamocolumnar junction is high.

Part B
Obstetrics

QUESTIONS

Medical disorders of pregnancy

1 A 26-year-old woman who is now 37 weeks' pregnant has been attending the antenatal clinic since she was 14 weeks. A routine full blood count performed by the midwife at 36 weeks is shown in Fig. 38.
a. What is the diagnosis?
b. What are the three reasons for the diagnosis?
c. What other symptoms may she present with?
d. What further investigation will you perform on her?

Fig. 38

e. What two treatment options may you recommend for her at this stage?

2 A young Afro-Carribean mother of two in her third pregnancy presented at 32 weeks' gestation with left upper abdominal pain and jaundice. Her haemoglobin is 8.7 g/dl. The uterus is soft and the fundal height is compatible with 30 weeks' gestation.
a. What two physical signs might you demonstrate to support a diagnosis of sickle cell anaemia?
b. What investigations will you perform to confirm the diagnosis?
c. What complication may she be having?

LEICESTERSHIRE HAEMATOLOGY SERVICE					Tel. ext: LRI 6530: LGH 4566: GGH 3575					
Consultant + Patient Loc. or GP Name + address			SURNAME				FORENAME			
			SEX F	DOB/AGE 26 years		HOSPITAL No.		LABORATORY No.		
Differential	Neutrophils	Lymphocytes	Monocytes	Eosinophils	Basophils	Atypical Lymph.	Metamyelo	Myelocytes	Pro. Mye	Blasts
WBC %	76.0	16.9	4.9	1.8	0.4					
x 10⁹/1	6.84	1.52	0.44	0.16	0.04					
% Adults Normal Range ABS	40-75 2.0-7.5	20-45 1.5-4.0	2-10 0.2-0.8	1-6 0.04-0.4	1 or less 0.01-0.1					
Machine Differential	Granulocytes	Lymphocytes	Mononuclears	WHITE CELL COMMENT						
WBC %										
	%	%	%							

Hb M 13.5-18.0 F 11.5-16.5	RBC M 4.5-6.5 F 3.9-5.6	HCT M 0.4-0.54 F 0.37-0.47	MCV 80-99	MCH 27 - 32	Reticulocytes 0 - 2	WBC 4 - 11	Platelets 150-400	P.V. 1.5-1.72	Date of Sample 13.07.97
8.2 g/dl	4.12 x 10¹²/1	0.252	68.4 fl	21.6 pg	%	9.0 x 10⁹/1	202 x 10⁹/1	cp	Date Reported 13.07.97 Run Page of

d. How will you confirm this?

e. What treatment will you offer her?

3 Mrs BYG is 32 weeks' pregnant in her third pregnancy. Her blood group is O rhesus D-negative while her husband is blood group A rhesus D-positive. Their other two children were not jaundiced at birth. She has developed rhesus antibodies at 32 weeks' gestation and is concerned about the effects of the antibodies on the fetus.

a. Why may she have developed antibodies this time?

b. Why might this baby not be affected?

c. What complications may occur *in utero* if the baby is not closely monitored and treatment offered where appropriate?

d. What complications may occur after delivery?

e. What treatment (if required) might be offered to the baby?

4 A primigravida is now 36 weeks' pregnant with rhesus D antibodies.

a. What four antenatal complications or procedures might have sensitized the mother?

b. The mother has been told that the fetus will require *in utero* blood transfusion. What blood group will be required for the transfusion?

c. How may the *in utero* transfusion be performed?

d. What will happen in the next pregnancy?

5 Mrs PB attended for routine antenatal care at 28 weeks' gestation when she was found to have + protein in her urine. She had no symptoms. An MSU grew *Escherichia coli* for which she was treated successfully. On two subsequent visits she was found to have proteinuria and an MSU showed significant bacterial growth but she remained asymptomatic.

a. What is this condition called?

b. What is the sequelae if this is untreated?

c. What two causes of this condition need to be excluded?

d. What treatment would this patient benefit from?

e. What further investigations need to be performed on her?

6 Mrs Bay had a renal transplant three years ago. She is on immunosuppressive therapy with azathioprine and is 20 weeks' pregnant.

a. What are the potential complications for this renal transplant patient in this pregnancy?

b. How will the patient be monitored in pregnancy?

c. How is the baby likely to be delivered?

d. Which contraceptive would you avoid in this patient?

7 A 27-year-old otherwise healthy primigravida attended the antenatal clinic at 32 weeks' gestation. A full blood count revealed a platelet count of 76 000/mm^3. A review of her notes showed that at booking her plaletelet count was 101 000/mm^3.

a. What is the most likely diagnosis of the condition?

b. What investigations would you like to perform on her?

c. What further tests do you need to perform to monitor the mother?

d. What precautions would you take during labour if the platelet count is less than 50 000/mm^3?

8 A 37-year-old woman in her third pregnancy has booked for antenatal care at 13 weeks' gestation She had severe pre-eclampsia and severe intrauterine growth retardation in her first pregnancy and was delivered at 34 weeks' gestation. Her second pregnancy was delivered at 35 weeks because of severe intrauterine growth retardation and oligohydramnios.

a. What is the likely medical cause of this woman's poor obstetric history.

b. What investigations may you perform to confirm your diagnosis?

c. What treatment might she be offered to improve the outcome of the pregnancy?

d. How may the pregnancy be monitored?

9 A 24-year-old woman with thyrotoxicosis is now 28 weeks' pregnant. She is taking carbimazole for her hyperthyroidism.

a. What are the effects of this disease on her pregnancy?

b. Which maternal investigation may predict the neonatal effect of this disease?

c. How does this affect the baby?

d. The mother attends your clinic at 36 weeks and complains of palpitations. What treatment would you recommend if she has tachycardia?

Fig. 39

e. How must the baby be monitored?

10 Mrs TO, who is 27 weeks' pregnant, has been told that she has a cardiac disease grade II.

a. What does cardiac disease grade II mean?

b. What are the effects of cardiac disease on pregnancy?

c. How should labour be managed?

d. If the mother has pulmonary hypertension, what advice will you offer her if she survives the pregnancy?

11 Molly is 23 years old and is in her first pregnancy. She presented at 32 weeks' gestation as an emergency with pruritus in the absence of dermatological abnormalities. A liver function test was performed and the result is shown in Fig. 39.

a. What is the likely diagnosis?

W360	LEICESTERSHIRE PATHOLOGY SERVICE CHEMICAL PATHOLOGY		
Cons/GP & Location:	UNIT NUMBER:		SURNAME:
	DoB/Age: 23 years	Sex: F	Forename:
	Patient Address:		
Specimen type:	Lab No:	Date & Time of report:	

Comment:

Diagnosis:

T. Bilirubin μmol/l 3-17	Alan. Trans. IU/l 2-53	Gamma G.T. IU/l 0-35f;50m	Alk. Phos. IU/l 40-130	Urate μmol/l 200,350f;500m	Phosphate mmol/l 0.8-1.4	T. protein g/l 60-80	Albumin g/l 35-55	Adj. Calcium mmol/l 2.1-2.6
15	69	33	220			65	37	

Sodium mmol/l 133-144	Potassium mmol/l 3.3-5.3	Bicarbonate mmol/l 22-30	Urea mmol/l 2.5-6.5	Creatinine μmol/l 60-120	Calcium mmol/l 2.1-2.6	Glucose mmol/l 4.0-6.6	Date & Time of Specimen	

QUOTED REFERENCE RANGES ARE FOR ADULTS

b. What other symptoms may she have presented with?

c. What other investigations must you perform?

d. What are the complications of this condition?

e. How may the pregnancy be managed?

12 A young girl was admitted into the medical ward at 36 weeks' gestation with vomiting, abdominal pain, jaundice and drowsiness. A liver function test showed elevated transaminases and phosphatases. A CT scan of the liver demonstrated fatty infiltration of the liver.

a. What is the most likely diagnosis?

b. What other three symptoms may she have had?

c. What are four possible complications of this condition?

d. How might the patient be managed?

e. Give four other causes of jaundice in pregnancy.

13 A 33-year-old known epileptic and her husband have come to see you for counselling. She is currently taking sodium valproate (Epilim) the only drug that will effectively control her fits. They would like to start a family.

a. What pre-pregnancy advice will you offer them?

b. What is the main complication of Epilim on the fetus?

c. What may happen when she becomes pregnant?

d. What factors may be responsible for the increase in drug requirements?

14 Miss LSE has been attending the rheumatology clinic because of recurrent joint pains, myalgia and weight loss. A blood test performed three months ago showed that she is positive for antinuclear antibody, anti-Ro/SSA antibody and anticardiolipin antibody. She is currently 12 weeks' pregnant.

a. What is the likely medical condition

this patient is suffering from?

b. What are the complications of this condition in pregnancy?

c. What treatment may be offered to reduce these complications?

d. How would you monitor the fetus?

15 A 17-year-old primigravida booked for antenatal care two weeks ago at eight weeks' gestation. Blood was taken for rubella antibody and the result came back as no antibodies detected. She has recently been in contact with a child who has German measles.

a. What are the potential risks of German measles to her baby?

b. What investigation might you perform to determine whether she might have been infected?

c. What symptoms might she have had?

d. If she was not infected, what measures will you take after delivery?

16 A mother of three who is 26 weeks' pregnant has been told that her three-year-old son has a disease called the 'slapped chick' or 'fifth' disease. She is very worried as her friend has told her that it may affect her baby.

a. What is responsible for this condition?

b. What symptoms may she have?

c. How may the infection reach the fetus?

d. What are the possible consequences of this infection on the fetus?

e. How may the diagnosis be confirmed?

17 An anxious nursery schoolteacher who is 20 weeks' pregnant has just been in contact with a toddler who has varicella-zoster (chickenpox) infection. She is unsure whether she herself has ever been infected with chickenpox.

a. What type of virus causes chickenpox?

b. How would you confirm that the mother has been infected before?

c. What are the complications of intrauterine chickenpox infection?

d. What are the main maternal complications of this infection in pregnancy?

e. If contact with the infected person occurred five days before delivery or within two days after birth, what additional precaution must be taken?

18 Mr and Mrs WM have recently returned from a holiday in France where they ate poorly cooked meat. Mrs WM is 18 weeks' pregnant and has recently read an article about toxoplasmosis in France. She has come to see you very concerned about this infection.

a. What is the causative organism for this infection?

b. What are the symptoms of this infection in adults?

c. What are the consequences of congenital toxoplasmosis?

d. How may you determine whether Mrs WM is infected or not?

e. How may the infection be treated?

f. How can infection with this organism be avoided?

19 Mrs PT is 29 weeks' pregnant and has recently returned from a holiday in the Carribean. She has been suffering from fever, chills, headaches and myalgia for the past three days. The fever is always worse in the evenings. Her GP found nothing abnormal on systemic examination. A viral screen was negative.

a. What is the likely cause of her pyrexia?

b. How would you confirm the diagnosis?

c. Which treatment will you recommend for her?

d. What are the possible complications of this condition if it is untreated?

20 A 26-year-old primigravida has been admitted as an emergency at 37 weeks' gestation having fitted at home. She has just had another fit.

a. What would be your initial management?

b. What four conditions may be responsible for the fits?

c. What four investigations would you perform to exclude some of these causes?

d. She has +++ protein in her urine but her blood pressure is only 100/70. Does that exclude eclampsia?

e. What will be your definite plan of management?

21 Mrs Abigail attended the antenatal clinic at 25 weeks' gestation and a routine urinalysis showed +++ glucose. A random blood glucose was performed (she last ate four hours ago) and the lab rang the result through. The level was 17 mmol/l.

a. What would be your next action?

b. Assuming that all these blood glucose levels are abnormal, what will be the diagnosis?

c. How will you manage and monitor the patient?

d. Why is urinary glucose not a reliable method of monitoring glycaemic control in pregnancy?

e. What other maternal complications must be excluded in this woman?

22 A young woman has been complaining of recurrent vulval boils in pregnancy. She is now 34 weeks and has been treated three time in this pregnancy for thrush infection.

a. What single important investigation would you like to perform on her?

b. What are six other indications for performing this test?

c. What are the common congenital malformations associated with diabetes mellitus?

d. When is the best time to deliver a diabetic patient in pregnancy?

23 A glucose tolerance test was performed on a woman who had a stillbirth at 39 weeks. The results are shown in Fig. 40.

a. What is the diagnosis?

W360			LEICESTERSHIRE PATHOLOGY SERVICE						
			CHEMICAL PATHOLOGY						

Cons/GP & Location: UNIT NUMBER: SURNAME:

DoB/Age: Sex: Forename:
33 years   F

Patient Address:

Specimen type: Blood   Lab No: Date & Time of report:

Fasting   = 5.5 mmol/1
60 minutes   = 12.4 mmol/1
120 minutes = 10.5 mmol/1

Comment:

Diagnosis:

T Bilirubin μmol/l 3-17	Alan. Trans. IU/l 2-53	Gamma G.T. IU/l 0-35f;50m	Alk. Phos. IU/l 40-130	Urate μmol/l 200,350f;500m	Phosphate mmol/l 0.8-1.4	T. protein g/l 60-80	Albumin g/l 35-55	Adj. Calcium mmol/l 2.1-2.6
Sodium mmol/l 133-144	Potassium mmol/l 3.3-5.3	Bicarbonate mmol/l 22-30	Urea mmol/l 2.5-6.5	Creatinine μmol/l 60-120	Calcium mmol/l 2.1-2.6	Glucose mmol/l 4.0-6.6	Date & Time of Specimen	

QUOTED REFERENCE RANGES ARE FOR ADULTS

Fig. 40

b. What treatment will you recommend for her?
c. What are the complications of the condition during pregnancy?
d. When is the baby most likely to be delivered?
e. If the mother is placed on insulin, what must be done soon after delivery?
f. What advice will you give this woman about the long-term implications of this condition?

24 This is a photograph (Fig. 41, see also colour plate section) of a baby delivered at 37 weeks' gestation by caesarean section.
a. What is the diagnosis?
b. What four complications is this baby likely to develop?
c. How might the cause of this condition

have been identified in the mother if it did not predate pregnancy?
d. What are the two most common intrapartum complications of this condition?

Hypertensive disorders of pregnancy

1 A 28-year-old primigravida is admitted onto the labour ward at 34 weeks' gestation with a blood pressure of 150/100 mmHg and +++ proteinuria. She booked at 12 weeks' gestation with a blood pressure of 110/60 and no proteinuria.
a. What is the likely diagnosis?
b. What five symptoms may she have?
c. What other four blood investigations would you like to perform?
d. What haematological complications may she develop?

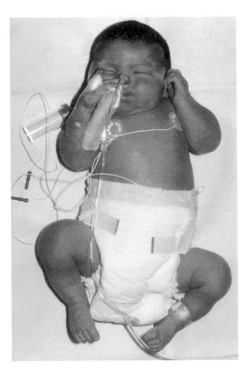

Fig. 41

2 The biochemistry report shown in Fig. 42 is on a blood sample obtained from a 35-year-old woman who presented to her midwife at 26 weeks' gestation
a. What are the abnormalities in the report?
b. What might have been the three indications for performing this test?
c. What two conditions may produce such abnormal biochemical results?
d. How may you distinguish between the two conditions?

3 Mrs AB complains of headaches, visual disturbances and nausea. She is 30 weeks' pregnant. A urinalysis showed ++++ protein and her blood pressure is 160/115 mmHg.
a. What does she have?
b. What are the possible five maternal complications of this condition if it is untreated?
c. How may she be managed?

d. What are four possible causes of maternal mortality in this condition?

4 Mrs Jones is planning on trying for a baby. She has come to see you for counselling about pre-eclampsia as her friend who is still in the renal unit with renal failure suffered from severe pre-eclampsia.
a. What are the risk factors for pre-eclampsia?
b. Can the occurrence of pre-eclampsia be predicted?
c. If she is high risk, can the disease be prevented?

5 A 17-year-old girl has been admitted at 31 weeks' gestation with pre-eclampsia.
a. What investigations will you perform on the fetus?
b. How will you monitor the mother?
c. What may be the fetal complications of this condition?
d. When would you like to deliver her?

6 A woman in her second pregnancy was admitted into the labour ward with right upper quadrant abdominal pain, severe headaches and blurred vision. A full blood count showed a haemoglobin of 10.2 g/dl despite the fact that her haemoglobin was 13.5 two weeks ago. The liver function test is shown in Fig. 43.
a. What is the diagnosis?
b. What does this means?
c. What other investigations would you like to perform?
d. What is the most appropriate management for this patient?

7 A women who was delivered by caesarean section because of pre-eclampsia has only been able to pass 30 ml of urine over the last four hours catheter in-situ and unblocked.
a. What may be the cause of this severe oliguria?

W360	LEICESTERSHIRE PATHOLOGY SERVICE		
	CHEMICAL PATHOLOGY		
Cons/GP & Location:	UNIT NUMBER:		SURNAME:
	DoB/Age: 35 years	Sex: F	Forename:
	Patient Address:		
Specimen type:	Lab No:		Date & Time of report:

Comment:

Diagnosis:

T. Bilirubin µmol/l 3-17	Alan. Trans. IU/l 2-53	Gamma G.T. IU/l 0-35f;50m	Alk. Phos. IU/l 40-130	Urate µmol/l 200,350f;500m	Phosphate mmol/l 0.8-1.4	T. protein g/l 60-80	Albumin g/l 35-55	Adj. Calcium mmol/l 2.1-2.6
10	28	32	50	350	1.0	61	34	

Sodium mmol/l 133-144	Potassium mmol/l 3.3-5.3	Bicarbonate mmol/l 22-30	Urea mmol/l 2.5-6.5	Creatinine µmol/l 60-120	Calcium mmol/l 2.1-2.6	Glucose mmol/l 4.0-6.6	Date & Time of Specimen
135	3.8	25	4.7	135	2.2		

QUOTED REFERENCE RANGES ARE FOR ADULTS

Fig. 42

b. How will you monitor her?
c. Why would such a patient develop anuria?
d. What is the course of this condition?

8 You were asked by the midwife to see a 32-year-old primigravida whose cooperation card is shown in Fig. 44.
a. What maternal condition has complicated this pregnancy?
b. State the probable effect of this condition on the fetus.
c. How will you confirm the diagnosis in the surgery?
d. What will be your next line of management?
e. What five investigations will you perform to monitor maternal well-being?

Antepartum and postpartum haemorrhage

1 The ultrasound photograph shown in Fig. 45 was taken from a grand multiparous woman at 36 weeks' gestation.
a. What does grand multiparous means?
b. What does the ultrasound photogaph show?
c. How may the woman have presented?
d. What is the main complication of this condition?
e. How may the baby be delivered

2 Figure 46 (see also colour plate section) was taken at delivery.
a. What does it show?
b. How might the woman have presented?
c. What signs may you elicit?
d. What are the maternal complications of this condition?

W360	LEICESTERSHIRE PATHOLOGY SERVICE							
	CHEMICAL PATHOLOGY							

Cons/GP & Location:

UNIT NUMBER:

SURNAME:

DoB/Age: 10.7.1962 Sex: F Forename:

Patient Address:

Specimen type: Lab No: Date & Time of report:

Comment:

Diagnosis:

T. Bilirubin µmol/l 3-17	Alan. Trans. IU/l 2-53	Gamma G.T. IU/l 0-35f;50m	Alk. Phos. IU/l 40-130	Urate µmol/l 200,350f;500m	Phosphate mmol/l 0.8-1.4	T. protein g/l 60-80	Albumin g/l 35-55	Adj. Calcium mmol/l 2.1-2.6
27	247		175			48	26	

Sodium mmol/l 133-144	Potassium mmol/l 3.3-5.3	Bicarbonate mmol/l 22-30	Urea mmol/l 2.5-6.5	Creatinine µmol/l 60-120	Calcium mmol/l 2.1-2.6	Glucose mmol/l 4.0-6.6	Date & Time of Specimen

QUOTED REFERENCE RANGES ARE FOR ADULTS

Fig. 43

3 Figure 47 shows a drug commonly used in most maternity units.
a. What is the drug called?
b. What is it used for?
c. When is it commonly given?
d. What does it prevent?
e. How can it be administered?
f. List three complications of this drug.
g. What are the three relative contraindications for its use?
h. What other two drugs may you use in its place?

4 A 29-year-old G5P4 is admitted as an emergency at 36 weeks' gestation with a history of sudden painless vaginal bleeding (losing approximately 200 ml). The pregnancy had hitherto been uncomplicated. Physical examination revealed the following: not pale, pulse 88/minute, blood pressure 105/65 mmHg, soft non-tender abdomen, fundal height 33 cm, single fetus lying transversely. The fetal heart rate was normal at 152/minute.
a. What is the most likely diagnosis?
b. What four reasons support your diagnosis?
c. What are your differential diagnoses?
d. What is your immediate management.
e. What further single investigation would you like to perform on her to confirm your diagnosis?

5 A 22-year-old woman in her second pregnancy is admitted at 38 weeks' gestation with constant lower abdominal pain associated with the passage of darkish blood and reduced fetal movements. On examination, her pulse is 100/minute and blood pressure 140/90. The symphysiofundal height is 38 cm but the

HOME VISIT BY MIDWIFE			INITIALS				U-S SCAN

EARLY DISCHARGE/FULL STAY PREFERRED

Treatment Remarks	Signature	Hb	Oes	H.P.L.	B.P.D. C.M.S.
M S U					
MSU sent.					
MSU — N AD					

SPECIAL POINTS (NB previous illnesses)	Blood Transfusion	V.D.R.L.
	Sheffield No.	Rub.A/b
	Blood Group	Rh.A/b
	Rhesus	S.C.Screen

PREFERRED HOSPITAL ....

PREFERRED CONSULTANT ....

ANTENATAL RECORD

Date	Amen. (Wks.)	Fundus	Pres. Pos.	Relation pp to Brim	F.H.	Urine Gluc.	Prot.	B.P.	Oed.	Weight kg.,	Return Visit. G.P.	Hosp.
26·6·97	9	—	—	—	—	NAD		110/60	—	63	5	
15·7·97	11+		—			N AD		120/65	—	64		35
30·7·97	14	14		—		NAD		125/70	—	67	4	
28·8·97	18	18	—	FM F	—	trace	—	110/75	—	70	4	
25·9·97	22	22	—		FHH with foetus	—	trace	120/70	—	73	4	
23·10·97	26	26	? ceph	FM F	FHHR	NAD		130/75	—	77	2	
5·11·97	28	27	Ceph	free	FHHR	NAD		120/80	+	80	2	
19·11·97	30	28	ceph	free	FHHR	—	trace	130/95	+	82	1	
26·11·97	31	28	ceph	free	FHHR	—	trace	135/85	+	83	/	
3·12·97	32	29	ceph	free	FHHR		+	145/95	++	86		

Menstrual History

Cycle	5/26–28	Date of last Cervical smear	12	6	94

Bleeding since LNMP 23 . 4 . 97

Date hormone tablets ceased

Years married | 1   Height 163 cm (NB >

FEEDING: BREAST | | BOTTLE | | UNCERTAIN

CHEST X-RAY | | | RESULT

DATE OF QUICKENING

Fig. 44

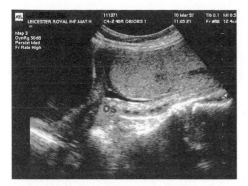

Fig. 45

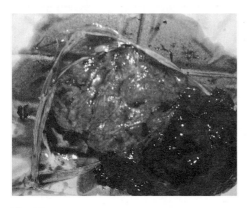

Fig. 46

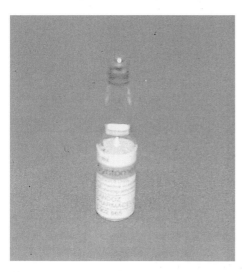

Fig. 47

uterus is tender and irritable. There is a single fetus with cephalic presentation and the head is engaged. The fetal heart is regular at 170/minute.

a. What is the most likely diagnosis?
b. What abdominal findings support your diagnosis?
c. What would be your immediate management?
d. When will you deliver the fetus?
e. How will you deliver the fetus?

6 The placenta in Fig. 48 (see also colour plate section) was delivered two hours ago.

a. What is wrong with it?
b. How may the patient present?
c. What important steps will you take to minimize these complications?
d. What three other lower genital tract conditions may present with postpartum haemorrhage?

7 You have been called to see a young woman at home who delivered 14 days ago in hospital. She had been experiencing a reddish discharge for the past week but in the last two days it has become heavy and bright red. Her uterus is still enlarged to about 16 weeks size.

a. What is the diagnosis?
b. What will your immediate management be?
c. What may be three causes of her bleeding?

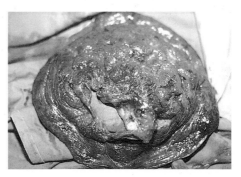

Fig. 48

d. Which three investigations will be performed in the hospital?
e. What treatment will she receive?

8 A young woman has just delivered following a significant placental abruption. Unfortunately, she has continued to bleed and her blood is no longer clotting.
a. What is the likely problem?
b. How will you diagnose the condition?
c. Which four other obstetric conditions may lead to the same problem?
d. How will coagulation be restored?

Prenatal diagnosis

1 A 27-year-old woman has come to book for antenatal care at 10 weeks' gestation.

Fig. 49

Her sister has a Down's syndrome child. She would like to discuss prenatal diagnosis.
a. What is the risk of her having a Down's syndrome child?
b. What is the blood test for Down's syndrome and how reliable is it?
c. Which definitive test can be performed at this gestation?
d. What are the disadvantages of this test?

2 This report shown in Fig. 49 is of a test performed on a 26-year-old primigravida at 17 weeks' gestation.
a. What is the correct interpretation of the test?
b. What three non-congenital conditions may be responsible for this result?
c. What single investigation can you perform to exclude most of these causes?
d. In the absence of any structural

W360	LEICESTERSHIRE PATHOLOGY SERVICE

CHEMICAL PATHOLOGY

Cons/GP & Location:	UNIT NUMBER:	SURNAME:

DoB/Age: 26	Sex: F	Forename:

Patient Address:

Specimen type: **Serum**   Lab No: Date & Time of report:

```
A-FETOPROTEIN    = 109 ug/l  (up to 68 ug/l)
Gestation        = 17 weeks
Free beta hCG    = 10.3 ug/l
AFP MoM          = 4.06
F-beta hCG MoM   = 1.17
Age at EDD       = 27
Down's Risk      = 1:1075
```

Comment:
Diagnosis:

T. Bilirubin μmol/l 3-17	Alan. Trans. IU/I 2-53	Gamma G.T. IU/I 0-35f;50m	Alk. Phos. IU/I 40-130	Urate μmol/l 200,350f;500m	Phosphate mmol/l 0.8-1.4	T. protein g/l 60-80	Albumin g/l 35-55	Adj. Calcium mmol/l 2.1-2.6

Sodium mmol/l 133-144	Potassium mmol/l 3.3-5.3	Bicarbonate mmol/l 22-30	Urea mmol/l 2.5-6.5	Creatinine μmol/l 60-120	Calcium mmol/l 2.1-2.6	Glucose mmol/l 4.0-6.6	Date & Time of Specimen	

QUOTED REFERENCE RANGES ARE FOR ADULTS

abnormalities, what other complications may she develop in this pregnancy?

3 This ultrasound photograph (Fig. 50) was taken from a 32-year-old G3P2 at 18 weeks' gestation.
a. What is the diagnosis?
b. What abnormal investigation may be suggestive of this condition?
c. What options are available to the mother?
d. What precautions may she take to reduce the recurrence risk of this abnormality?

4 Anterior abdominal wall defects are not uncommon. The outcome is said to depend on the type of defect and the centre (hospital) where the baby is born.
a. What are the two most common anterior abdominal wall defects that you may encounter?
b. What are the differences between the two?
c. How will prenatal counselling differ in the two conditions?
d. What other biochemical test may be abnormal in these women?

5 The report shown in Fig. 51 belongs to your patient who is 15 weeks' pregnant and is coming to see you for discussion.
a. What does it show?
b. What two options are available to her?

c. She has decided to undergo an invasive test. What are the differences between the two common tests available?
d. Can ultrasound diagnose Down's syndrome?

6 A couple have come to see you for counselling about prenatal diagnosis because they are both carriers of a cystic fibrosis gene.
a. What are the chances of their offspring being affected?
b. How may a diagnosis be made prenatally?
c. What other antenatal clinical manifestations of cystic fibrosis may be identified on ultrasound scan?
d. How early may the prenatal diagnostic test be performed?

7 A 19-year-old primigravida came for an anomaly scan at 18 weeks' gestation because the maternal serum alpha-fetoprotein levels were raised (more than 2.5 times the median).
a. What four fetal malformations may cause a high maternal serum alpha-fetoprotein?
b. She has had an ultrasound scan and the fetus has anencephaly. What will be the clinical presentation of this condition in late pregnancy?
c. Why will an anencephalic fetus present this way?
d. In the presence of anencephaly, why may pregnancy be prolonged?

8 Mrs B is a 25-year-old primigravida who presented for a blood test for Down's syndrome. She had an ultrasound scan at booking which showed a single pregnancy and also agreed with her dates. She was visited by her midwife yesterday who revealed that her blood test (Fig. 52) was abnormal. She is very upset and has come to see you for counselling and further management. At 25 years her age-related risk for Down's syndrome is 1 : 1350.

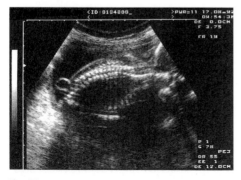

Fig. 50

W360	LEICESTERSHIRE PATHOLOGY SERVICE CHEMICAL PATHOLOGY		

Cons/GP & Location:	UNIT NUMBER:		SURNAME:
	DoB/Age: 13.08.1961	Sex: F	Forename:
	Patient Address:		

Specimen type: Serum	Lab No:	Date & Time of report: 12.05.97 15:13

```
A-FOETOPROTEIN    = 10 KU/L      (up to 51)
GESTATION (SCAN)  = 15 WEEKS
Free-Beta hCG     = 28.5 UG/L
AFP MoM           = 0.37
F-B hCG MoM       = 1.72
AGE AT EDD        = 36 YEARS
DOWN'S RISK 1 in  = 50           (101 to 32000)
```

Comment:
Diagnosis: LMP: 17.1.97, EDD 26.10.97 IDD/PVB NO (R)

T Bilirubin µmol/l 3-17	Alan. Trans. IU/l 2-53	Gamma G.T. IU/l 0-35f;50m	Alk. Phos. IU/l 40-130	Urate µmol/l 200,350f;500m	Phosphate mmol/l 0.8-1.4	T. protein g/l 60-80	Albumin g/l 35-55	Adj. Calcium mmol/l 2.1-2.6

Sodium mmol/l 133-144	Potassium mmol/l 3.3-5.3	Bicarbonate mmol/l 22-30	Urea mmol/l 2.5-6.5	Creatinine µmol/l 60-120	Calcium mmol/l 2.1-2.6	Glucose mmol/l 4.0-6.6	Date & Time of Specimen	

QUOTED REFERENCE RANGES ARE FOR ADULTS

Fig. 51

a. Which two biochemical abormalities are associated with Down's syndrome?
b. What is the implication of this result?
c. What further advice will you give this woman?
d. How reliable are these two tests?

9 Mrs LFC is a 32-year-old housewife who had a termination for Down's syndrome two years ago. She is pregnant again but this time she has twins. A booking ultrasound scan at 10 weeks' gestation agrees with her dates. She is very anxious about having another Down's syndrome fetus.

a. What is the risk of either of her fetuses being affected?
b. She has been told by a friend that an ultrasound scan around 12 weeks may identify a fetus with Down's syndrome. What exactly is this test?
c. Could she have the blood test for Down's syndrome?
d. Which test can she definitely have to determine if she is carrying an affected baby?
e. What are the problems with this test in her case?
f. If it was possible to define the affected fetus with some certainty, what two options may she have?

10 A Nigerian couple have come to see you because they would like to have a second child. The husband is rhesus-positive and the wife is rhesus-negative. Their first child, delivered in their country, has sickle cell anaemia (HbSS) and they do not want to have another affected child. They are concerned about the risk of having another child with

W360	LEICESTERSHIRE PATHOLOGY SERVICE			
	CHEMICAL PATHOLOGY			

Cons GP & Location:	UNIT NUMBER:		SURNAME:
	DoB/Age: 25 years	Sex: F	Forename:
	Patient Address:		

Specimen type: Serum   Lab No: Date & Time of report: 27.01.1998

Alpha-foetoprotein (AFP)	= 15 ku/l
AFP MoM	= 0.56
Free-Beta hCG	= 79.6 ug/l
Free-beta hCG MoM	= 4.80
Gestation by scan	= 15 weeks
Age at EDD	= 25 years
Down's risk 1 in	= 33
AFP Median	= *27.0 ku/l
Free-Beta hCG Median	= *16.6 ug/l
AFP 95th centile	= 51

Comment:
Diagnosis: LMP 13.10.97, EDD 29.07.98

T Bilirubin µmol/l 3-17	Alan. Trans. IU/l 2-53	Gamma G.T. IU/l 0-35f;50m	Alk. Phos. IU/l 40-130	Urate µmol/l 200,350f;500m	Phosphate mmol/l 0.8-1.4	T. protein g/l 60-80	Albumin g/l 35-55	Adj. Calci. mmol/l 2.1-2.6

Sodium mmol/l 133-144	Potassium mmol/l 3.3-5.3	Bicarbonate mmol/l 22-30	Urea mmol/l 2.5-6.5	Creatinine µmol/l 60-120	Calcium mmol/l 2.1-2.6	Glucose mmol/l 4.0-6.6	Date & Time of Specime

QUOTED REFERENCE RANGES ARE FOR ADULTS

Fig. 52

sickle cell anaemia and have a few questions for you.

a. Why is the child affected when neither of the parents are affected?
b. What are the chances of their next baby being affected?
c. What pre-pregnancy investigation must they have if it has not already been performed?
d. What prenatal investigation will you offer them?
e. List two complications of this test.

Fetal monitoring

1 A woman has just been to hospital at 41 weeks' gestation and was given the form shown in Fig. 53.

a. What is it called?
b. When would you give someone this chart? (Give three indications for its use.)
c. What instructions will you give the woman?
d. If she reports to the hospital with reduced or absent fetal movements, what investigation would you like to perform?

2 The ultrasound scan report below was obtained from a 27-year-old G2P1 at 29 weeks' gestation. She was well and fetal movements were considered to be normal. *Ultrasound report:* Single active fetus, cephalic presentation. Placenta is fundal and anterior. Reduced liquor volume. BPD = 60 mm = 28 weeks, HC = 178 mm = 29 weeks, AC = 140 mm = 25 weeks, FL = 25 mm = 28 weeks. Fetal kidneys, stomach and bladder seen.

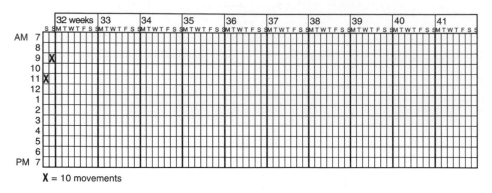

Fig. 53

a. What is the diagnosis?
b. What three conditions may be responsible for this condition?
c. How will the pregnancy be monitored from now onwards? (Give three methods of monitoring.)
d. What will determine the time the baby will be delivered?

3 The cardiotocogram (CTG) shown in Fig. 54 was taken from a 26-year-old woman who presented at 38 weeks' gestation with reduced fetal movements.
a. What abnormalities are shown on the CTG?
b. What will be the most likely plan of management?
c. Further CTGs show persistence of this pattern. What will you advise?
d. If she went into labour, what must you do?

4 A young woman in her second pregnancy has just been to the hospital where she has been told that her baby needs close monitoring because she is hypertensive and the baby is small for gestational age. She had a biophysical profile performed and Doppler studies of the fetal umbilical artery.

a. What is involved in a biophysical profile?
b. At her next visit, she is told that the Doppler is abnormal. What may be regarded as an abnormal Doppler waveform?
c. How else can her baby be monitored?
d. She delivers a 1.8 kg baby at 38 weeks' gestation. What are the four neonatal complications for this baby?
e. Are there any long-term complications of this condition for the baby? (Give three.)

5 A schoolteacher has come to your antenatal clinic at 42 weeks' gestation. She is aware of the fact that women are induced at 42 weeks' gestation but she would prefer to go as far as possible. She is, however, concerned about fetal monitoring.
a. How may her baby be monitored?
b. What are the three likely complications of post-maturity?
c. She decides after three days of monitoring to be induced. She has been assessed and told that her Bishop's score is 4. What constitutes a Bishop's score?
d. How may she be induced assuming the cervix is closed?

6 The cooperation card shown in Fig. 55 belongs to a primigravida who is now 38 weeks. She is well and her fetal movements are described as normal.

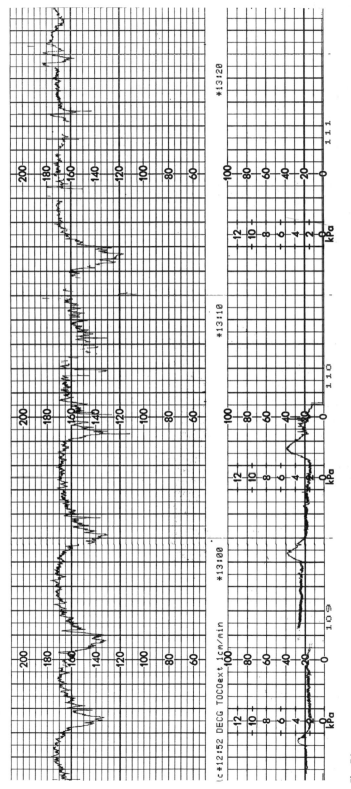

Fig. 54

	PREFERRED HOSPITAL					ANTENATAL RECORD						
	PREFERRED CONSULTANT											
Date	Amen. (Wks.)	Fundus	Pres. Pos.	Relation pp to Brim	F.H.	Urine Gluc.	Urine Prot.	B.P.	Oed.	Weight kg.,	Return Visit G.P.	Return Visit Hosp.
28·4·95	12	—		—		NAD		110/60		70	4	
12	14					NAD		110/70	—	72		35
25·5·95	16	16		—		NAD		110/75		75	4	
23·6·95	20	20		—	—	NAD		120/70		75	4	
20·7·95	24	24		—	—	+		120/70		78	8	
10·8·95	28	26	ceph	free	H	NAD		120/80		78		41
14·9·95	32	30	breech	free	H	NAD		130/70		79	2	
23·9·95	34	31cm	ceph	free	H	NAD		120/80		80	2	
13·10·95	36	32	ceph	free	H	—	Nil testH	125/75		78	2	

Menstrual History   6/28

Cycle | Date of last Cervical smear 3/10/95

Bleeding since LNMP   'nil'

Date hormone tablets ceased

Years married 3   Height 5'7" cm (NB >

FEEDING: BREAST | BOTTLE | UNCERTAIN

CHEST X-RAY | RESULT

DATE OF QUICKENING

HOME VISIT BY MIDWIFE [   ] INITIALS
EARLY DISCHARGE/FULL STAY PREFERRED

Treatment Remarks	Signature	Hb	Oes	H.P.L.	B.P.D. C.M.S.
Random glucose 4·5 mmol/L Well. Going on.					
well good fh.					

U·S SCAN

SPECIAL POINTS (NB previous illnesses)
    Smokes 20-30/day

Blood Transfusion		V.D.R.L.	Neg
Sheffield No.		Rub.A/b	+ve.
Blood Group	O	Rh.A/b	
Rhesus	D +ve.	S.C.Screen	

Fig. 55

a. What is the possible abnormality from the card?
b. What investigation will you request to confirm your diagnosis?
c. What particular aspects of this investigation will you be interested in?
d. What other three investigations may you perform on the baby once your diagnosis is confirmed?
e. What are the prenatal complications of this condition?

7 A 21-year-old primigravida is seen for antenatal follow-up at 38 weeks' gestation when the fundal height is measured to be 34 cm. There is a single fetus lying longitudinally with cephalic presentation.
a. What is the most likely diagnosis?
b. What investigation would you perform to confirm your diagnosis?
c. What information do you expect from this test?
d. How may you monitor the baby?
e. What are the fetal consequences of this condition?

Preterm labour and premature rupture of fetal membranes

1 A 25-year-old woman in her third pregnancy presented at 30 weeks' gestation with a history suspicious of premature rupture of fetal membranes.
a. How might you confirm the diagnosis of ruptured membranes?
b. If the membranes have indeed ruptured, what are the risks of the complication?
c. You have decided to manage the patient conservatively. How will you monitor the pregnancy?
d. What is the main danger of premature labour?
e. How can the severity of this complication be reduced?

2 Mrs AO is booking for antenatal care in her fourth pregnancy at 12 weeks'

gestation. The first pregnancy ended in a preterm labour at 26 weeks' gestation and the baby died of extreme prematurity. The second was delivered at 28 weeks' gestation. Although the baby also suffered from respiratory distress syndrome he is, however, alive and well. The third was lost at 18 weeks' gestation. She had noticed a certain gush of water and by the time she had arrived at the hospital, the baby had already been delivered.
a. What is the most likely cause of the preterm labours in this patient?
b. How may this be diagnosed in pregnancy?
c. What treatment may be offered to her and when?
d. If such a treatment is offered, what will be the indications for discontinuing it?
e. In the absence of any complications what will be the best time to discontinue the treatment?

3 Mrs Taylor is a solicitor in her second pregnancy. Her daughter was admitted into the neonatal unit with beta-haemolytic *Streptoccocus* infection two days after delivery. She had had a high vaginal swab at 28 weeks' gestation for a vaginal discharge but was not treated despite the isolation of beta-haemolytic *Streptoccocus*. She is now 32 weeks and is concerned about this infection.
a. How common is this organism?
b. What will be the plan for this pregnancy?
c. What if the fetal membranes rupture?
d. What if she goes into labour before any treatment is offered to her?
e. What will happen to her baby at this time?

4 Preterm labour is the most common cause of perinatal mortality and morbidity.
a. What investigations would you perform on a woman presenting with preterm labour at 31 weeks' gestation?
b. What may be the four causes of preterm labour in such a patient?

c. Which two drugs might you give to stop the contractions?
d. What are three possible maternal side-effects of these drugs?
e. What is the main complication of combining one of these drugs with steroids and intravenous fluids?

5 A 32-year-old G3P1 presented at 30 weeks' gestation with regular uterine contractions (occurring every 4–5 minutes). There was no associated vaginal bleeding or spontaneous rupture of the fetal membranes. The cervix was 2 cm dilated and fetal membranes were felt to be intact.
a. What is the diagnosis?
b. What three investigations would you perform on her?
c. Give four fetal/neonatal complications of this condition.
d. How will you reduce the incidence of one of these complications?
e. Which drugs can be administered to stop or delay delivery?

Labour (normal and abnormal)

1 Mrs BRI is a primigravida who was admitted in labour at 39 weeks' gestation. Her cervix was 3 cm dilated and fetal membranes were intact. She was having 3–4 contractions every 10 minutes. The contractions were described as strong and lasting for 30–45 seconds. The admission CTG was normal. Four hours later, she was examined and the cervix was still 3 cm.
a. What is the diagnosis?
b. What steps will you take to rectify the labour?
c. Two hours later, the contractions are infrequent and short-lasting. What would be your next step?
d. Four hours later (after regular strong and frequent contractions), she is only 5 cm. What would suggest that there may be fetopelvic disproportion?

e. How will this obstruction be overcome?

2 A woman who delivered 30 minutes ago has just collapsed.
a. What will be your initial management?
b. Apart from uterine inversion what are four other possible causes of the collapse?
c. What other three signs may a woman with uterine inversion have?
d. What is the definitive treatment of this condition in (c)?

3 You are called to see a woman who started bleeding profusely soon after the placenta was delivered.
a. What would be your first line of management?
b. What would be your next line of management?
c. What may be responsible for this complication?
d. The placenta and membranes are complete and there is no trauma from the lower genital tract but she is still continuing to bleed. What will be your next line of management?

4 A woman was admitted into the delivery suite at 38 weeks' gestation with absent fetal movements for 24 hours and the fetal heart could not be picked up with the CTG machine.
a. How will you confirm the diagnosis of intrauterine fetal death?
b. What will your immediate management be?
c. What investigations would you perform on the mother?
d. What three investigations might you perform on the fetus?
e. What two investigations would you perform on the placenta?

5 A 42-year-old G6P5 (all previous full-term normal deliveries) has come to see you at 37 weeks' gestation because she wants a home confinement.

a. Why may it not be safe for her to deliver at home?
b. What are the complications that you are worried about?
c. She decides to have a home confinement but fails to go into labour by 42 weeks. The baby is also clinically larger than her last five babies. Why would you prefer her to deliver in the hospital?
d. What other advice would you offer after she has delivered?

6 A woman who had an emergency caesarean section in her first pregnancy went into spontaneous labour at 39 weeks. Labour was progressing normally until the fetal heart rate dropped suddenly. A diagnosis of ruptured uterus was made.
a. What other clinical features will support this diagnosis?
b. What is the immediate management?
c. The rupture has been repaired successfully. Will you sterilize the patient?
d. How would a subsequent pregnancy be delivered?
e. If she had a classic scar on her uterus, when is it more likely to rupture?

7 Mrs K has cardiac disease grade II. She was admitted in labour at 41 weeks.
a. What extra precautions must you take in the first stage?
b. What must you not do in the second stage?
c. What precautions might you take in the second stage?
d. Why is it dangerous to administer fast-acting oxytocics?

Multiple pregnancy, polyhydramnios and oligohydramnios

1 Mrs A, who is a twin, presented to the antenatal clinic at 28 weeks' gestation in her fourth pregnancy. She booked at 12 weeks' gestation by her dates when a booking scan was performed. The symphysiofundal height measured 44 cm and fetal parts were difficult to palpate. The fetal heart rate was, however, heard with a sonicaid.
a. What additional information about her booking ultrasound scan will help in making the diagnosis?
b. What are the possible causes of the significantly large fundal height?
c. What two important investigations would you like to perform on her?
d. Give six potential complications of this pregnancy?

2 Figure 56 is an ultrasound photograph taken at 16 weeks' gestation from a 32-year-old woman.
a. What is the diagnosis?
b. What clinical features may lead to a suspicion of this condition?
c. What are the maternal antenatal complications of this condition?
d. What are the fetal complications of this condition?

3 Mrs XY went into spontaneous labour at 36 weeks' gestation for a clomiphene-induced twin pregnancy. She had taken clomiphene citrate for 16 months.
a. What are three second stage complications of this condition in labour?

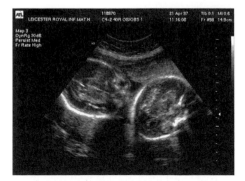

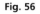
Fig. 56

b. What is the most common third stage complicaton?

c. How will you prevent this third stage complicaton?

d. What is the main risk of giving the mother prolonged clomiphene therapy?

4 An ultrasound scan performed on a 26-year-old multiparous woman because of suspected small for gestational age is shown below. A booking ultrasound scan at 14 weeks had not revealed any abnormality and her dates had agreed with ultrasound dates.

Ultrasound scan report: Single active fetus. BPD = 216 mm = 34 weeks, HC = 247 mm = 33 weeks, AC = 216 mm = 32 weeks, FL = 32 mm = 34 weeks. There is anhydramnios. The fetal bladder and kidneys have not been visualized; however, the anhydramnios might have made this difficult.

a. What is the meaning of anhydramnios?

b. What important question must you ask the woman?

c. What are three possible causes of this problem?

d. What are the consequences of this condition on the fetus?

e. What advice will you give the woman?

5 A 35-year-old woman has just been told at booking that she has twins. She is very worried about zygosity as she has been told that there are two types, one of which is associated with a greater risk of complications.

a. Which type of twins are associated with a greater risk of complications?

b. How can this be diagnosed at booking?

c. What complications are more likely in a monozygotic twin pregnancy?

d. How may twin-to-twin transfusion be identified antenatally?

e. What options are available for managing twin-to-twin transfusion?

6 Mrs G is a primigravida who went for a growth scan at 28 weeks because the fundal height was much larger than her dates. The report states that there is polyhydramnios and a double bubble appearance within the fetal abdomen.

a. What is the most likely diagnosis?

b. What chromosomal abnormality may be associated with such a finding?

c. How may this be excluded?

d. What other abnormalities may present with a double bubble appearance in the fetal abdomen?

7 A 28-year-old multigravida with a singleton pregnancy presnted at 30 weeks with a three-day history of a rapidly enlarging abdomen, difficulties with breathing when lying flat and very swollen legs and vulva. The symphysiofundal height was 36 cm and the abdomen was shiny and fetal parts were difficult to palpate.

a. What is the diagnosis?

b. What four fetal conditions may give rise to the condition in this patient?

c. Which single clinical sign may you demonstrate?

d. How may the cardiorespiratory compromise be alleviated?

e. What is the drawback of this procedure?

f. What drug could be used to improve the condition?

g. What are two possible side-effects of this drug on the fetus?

8 Mrs Gordon has conceived after her third IVF attempt. She has just had an ultrasound scan at six weeks and has been told that she has triplets.

a. What three possible first trimester complications may she have?

b. What prophylactic drugs must she have during pregnancy?

c. What would be the most common complication in the second half of pregnancy?

d. What three other maternal complications may arise?

e. What precautions might be taken to

reduce the risk and complications of prematurity?

f. How may the babies be delivered?

Instrumental delivery

1 The instrument shown in Fig. 57 is commonly used on the labour ward.

a. What is the name of the instrument?

b. In which three situations may it be used?

c. What six conditions must be fulfilled before the application of this instrument?

d. What four complications may arise from the use of this instrument?

2 Figure 58 shows an instrument used in obstetrics.

a. What is the instrument?

b. What are the indications for its use?

c. What are the possible complications of this instrument

d. When will it be advantageous to use this instrument rather than a forceps?

e. What are the contraindications for using this instrument?

3 Figure 59 shows a set of instruments?

a. What are the instruments used for?

b. What abnormal fetal heart rate patterns would necessitate the use of these instruments?

c. What may be responsible for a false abnormal reading from this test?

d. What type of reading would you act on?

e. Why is this test necessary despite the use of fetal heart rate tracing?

4 Identify each of the instruments in Fig. 60 and give an indication for its use and a complication.

Puerperium

1 You have been called to see a 34-year-old woman with a temperature of 38.7 °C six days after an emergency caesarean section.

a. What five symptoms may she have?

b. What five specific clinical signs may you demonstrate?

c. What five investigations might you perform?

d. What are the five possible causes of her pyrexia?

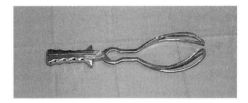

Fig. 57

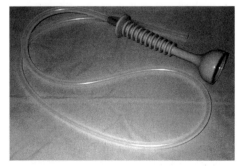

Fig. 58

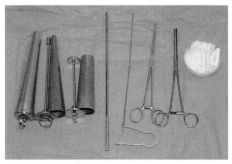

Fig. 59

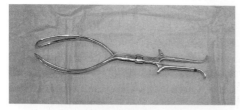

(a)

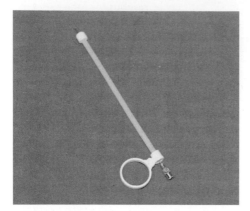

(b)

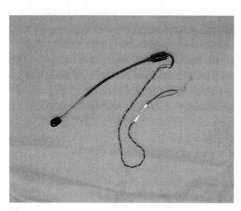

(c)

Fig. 60

a. What is the most likely diagnosis?
b. How will you confirm your diagnosis?
c. What treatment will you offer her?
d. What five factors increase the risk of deep venous thrombosis in pregnancy?
e. What investigations might you perform on anyone with a risk factor for deep venous thrombosis?

3 A young 17-year-old who delivered her first baby four days ago has been observed by the midwife to be weepy, anxious and irritable. Pregnancy and labour had been uncomplicated.
a. What is the most likely diagnosis?
b. What other two symptoms may she have?
c. What investigation(s) may you perform?
d. What would your management be?
e. When is it likely to progress to postnatal depression?

4 Mrs HG delivered two weeks ago following an uncomplicated pregnancy. Three years ago, she had a nervous breakdown at work and was treated for depression. She now exhibits an inability to love her baby and, in addition, has become suicidal and very withdrawn.
a. What is the most likely diagnosis?
b. What other three symptoms may she present with?
c. What would be your immediate management?
d. What treatment will she be offered?
e. What other medical condition may you wish to exclude?

2 You are called to see an obese woman who experienced a sudden chest pain 10 days after a forceps delivery. A chest X-ray is reported as normal but her ECG shows some evidence of right ventricular strain. Her blood gases are reported as: PaO_2 7.6 kPa, $PaCO_2$ 4.1 kPa.

5 The chart shown in Fig. 61 is that of a mother who delivered seven days ago. She has been breast feeding succcessfully. On examination, she does not have any chest signs, abdominal tenderness or abnormal vaginal discharge. The uterus is well involuted and the lochia is normal. Her legs are not swollen and her urine MSU is negative.

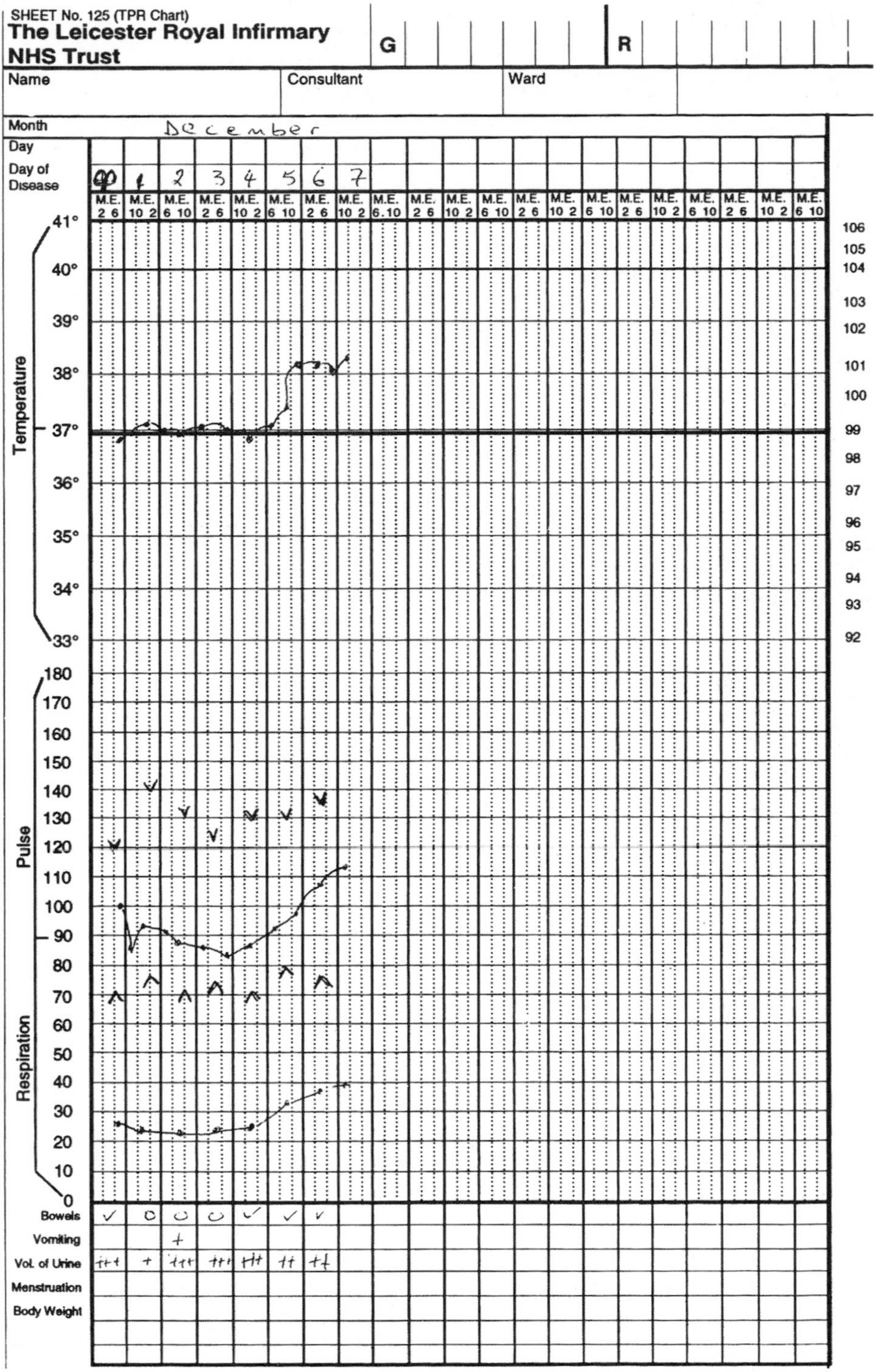

SHEET No. 125 (TPR Chart)
The Leicester Royal Infirmary
NHS Trust

Month	December

Day of Disease: 90, 1, 2, 3, 4, 5, 6, 7

Temperature axis: 41° to 33° (°C) / 106 to 92 (°F)

Pulse axis: 180 to 0
Respiration axis: 90 to 10

Bowels	✓	0	0	0	✓	✓	✓
Vomiting		+					
Vol. of Urine	+++	+	+++	+++	+++	++	++
Menstruation							
Body Weight							

Fig. 61

a. What may be the other source of her temperature?
b. What other two symptoms may she have?
c. What three localized signs would you look for?
d. How will you manage her?

6 You have been asked by a midwife to see a young woman who delivered six days ago and whose episiotomy has broken down. You have examined her and the episiotomy site is necrotic and is discharging a foul-smelling copius yellowish discharge.
a. What will be your immediate management?
b. What advice would you give the woman?
c. What advice will you give the midwife?
d. What is the long-term management of this patient?

7 Mrs MM has been discharged home following the delivery of a stillborn at 35 weeks' gestation.
a. How may Mrs MM's lactation be suppressed?
b. What is the major disadvantage of using drugs to suppress lactation in this case?
c. What advice must you give the couple if you are to place the woman on this drug?
d. How long will it take for menstruation to resume?

8 A woman who delivered eight weeks ago and is not breast feeding is yet to menstruate. She has come to see you about this and the only information you have been able to obtain from her is that she had very severe primary postpartum haemorrhage.
a. What is the most likely diagnosis?
b. What is the pathophysiology of this condition?
c. What other two symptoms may she present with?

d. What three hormonal investigations would you perform to confirm the diagnosis?
e. How may she be managed?

Abnormal lie and presentation

1 A 27-year-old gravida 2 was seen by the midwife at 38 weeks' gestation with a suspected breech presentation.
a. What four factors may be responsible for this abnormal presentation?
b. What single investigation will you perform to confirm your diagnosis?
c. What other information would you like from the investigation?
d. What are the dangers of a breech labour?
e. What other investigation would you like to perform before discussing delivery options with this woman?

2 Mrs B is 38 weeks in her third pregnancy. She has just been to the antenatal clinic to see you and you have found that the baby is lying obliquely. Three days ago she had seen the midwife who noted the fetus to be in a transverse positon.
a. What is the diagnosis?
b. What would you like to exclude in this pregnancy?
c. What are the main complications of this condition?
d. What will be the most likely course of action?
e. What is likely to happen on the ward?

3 A primiparous woman had an ultrasound scan at 10 weeks' gestation and was told that she had a large fibroid in the posterior wall of the uterus. She has not had any symptoms associated with the fibroid but is concerned about the consequences of the fibroid in this pregnancy.
a. What are the possible complications of the fibroid in pregnancy?
b. At 35 weeks, she presents with a

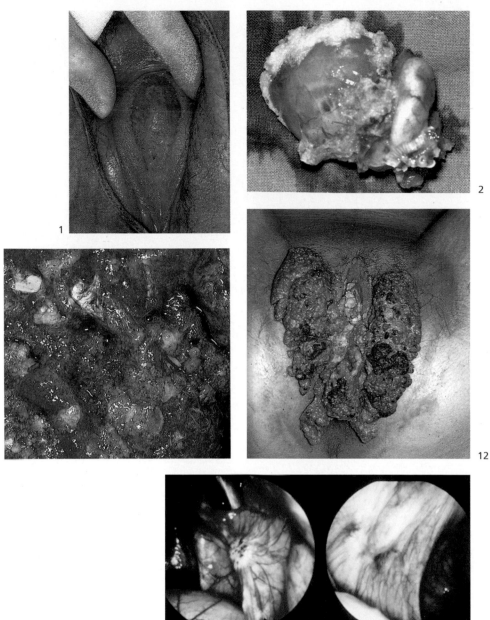

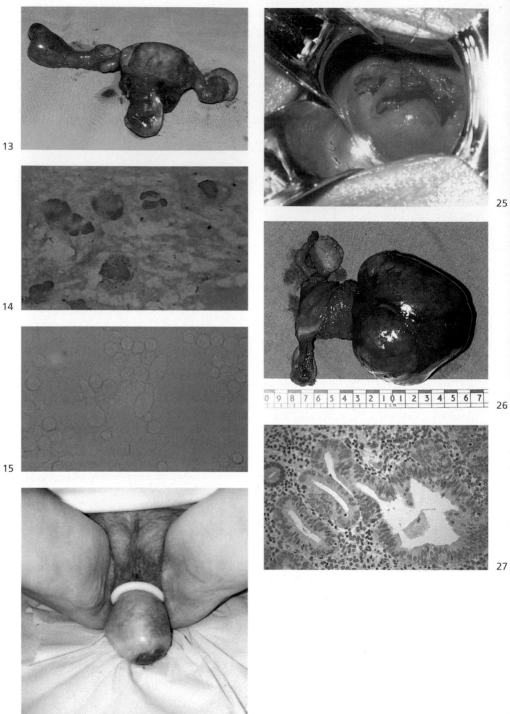

13

14

15

19

25

26

27

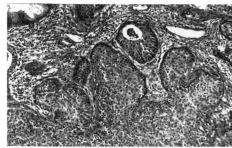

29a

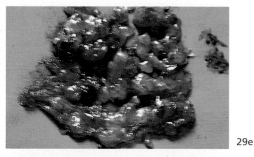

29e

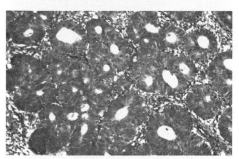

29b

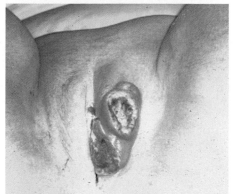

30

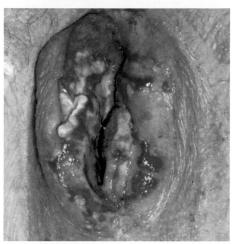

29c

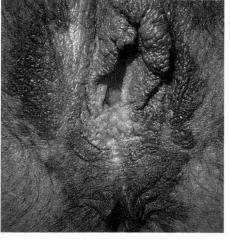

31

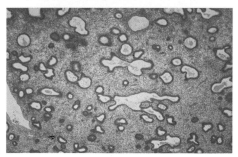

29d

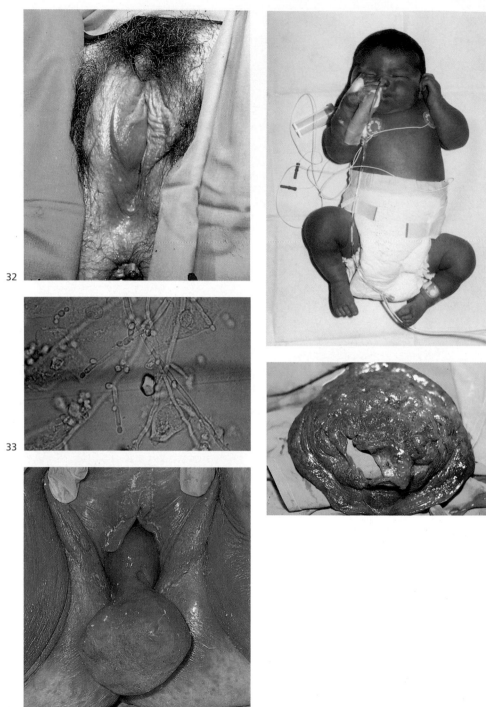

32

33

34

41 &
66

48

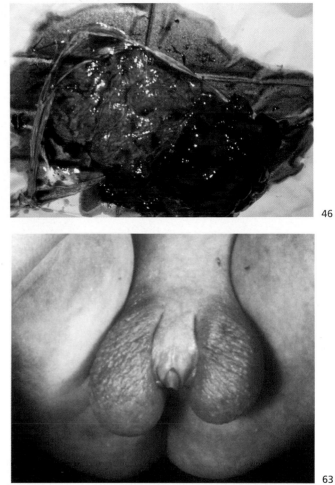

46

63

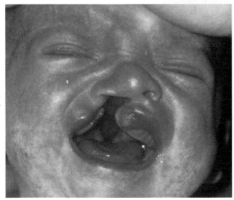

68

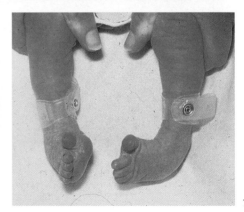

77

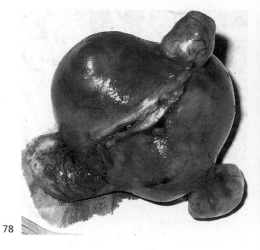

78

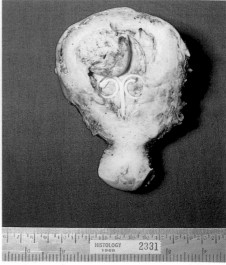

2331

97

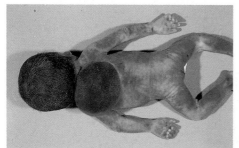

88

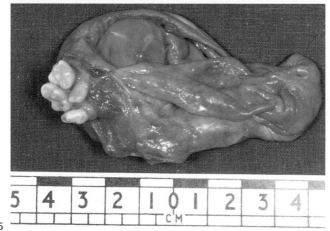

96

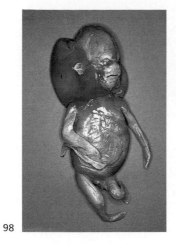

98

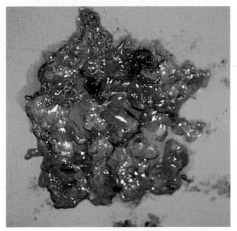

99

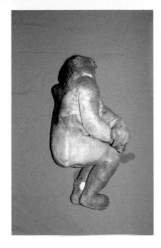

100

transverse fetus. What investigation must you perform and why?

c. The fetus remains in the transverse position at 39 weeks. How will you deliver it?

d. How will the fibroid be managed in pregnancy?

Drugs in pregnancy

1 Mrs DD is 26 weeks' pregnant and presented with a profuse vaginal discharge for one week. A high vaginal swab was reported as showing *Gardnerella vaginalis*, mixed anaerobes and *Bacteroides* species.

a. What treatment will you recommend for her (dose and duration of treatment)?

b. What are the side-effects of this drug?

c. If she does not take the treatment, what may the consequences be on the pregnancy?

2 A young girl who is 10 weeks' pregnant developed a deep venous thrombosis while on the pill and was subsequently placed on warfarin which she is still taking.

a. What are the teratogenic effects of warfarin?

b. What is the best management for her?

c. What important investigation will you perform later in pregnancy?

d. For how long will you maintain her on the alternate treatment?

e. Are there any side-effects of this treatment?

3 A pregnant women presented at 38 weeks' gestation with a creamy vaginal discharge. An endocervical swab revealed *Neisseria gonorrhoeae*. She went into labour before treatment could be instituted.

a. What treatment would you recommend for this woman?

b. What is the risk of this infection to the neonate?

c. If the baby is infected, when will it manifest symptoms?

d. What symptom may the neonate exhibit?

e. What treatment will you recommend for the baby?

f. What additional step must you take?

Activity stations

1 This is a urine sample obtained from a woman at 28 weeks' gestation. Test the urine and answer the following questions (candidate needs to identify protein).

a. What is present in the urine?

b. What could be responsible for the presence of this substance in the urine?

c. What further investigations would you like to carry out?

2 A woman attending for ANC at 30 weeks gestation produced this urine sample (sample contains nitrates which the candidate has to identify on testing).

a. What is present in the urine?

b. What could be the cause of this?

c. What investigation will you perform?

d. If the woman is not treated (as she is asymptomatic) what complications may arise?

3 A woman attending for ANC at 30 weeks gestation produced this urine sample (sample contains glucose which the candidate has to identify on testing).

a. What does your urinalysis show?

b. What further investigation would you like to perform on her?

c. If the result is abnormal, what would be your next line of management?

d. What are the main complications of this condition in late pregnancy?

4 Frances is a 22-year-old single unemployed woman at 20 weeks gestation presenting with a thick yellowish vaginal discharge and dysuria six days after meeting her new partner. She has a history

of pelvic inflammatory disease and has had four sexual partners in the last six months. What would you do?

Interactive questions

1 This 24-year-old G2P1 had a termination of pregnancy for Down's syndrome at 18 weeks' gestation two years ago. She is currently eight weeks' pregnant and has come to see you for counselling about prenatal diagnosis.
During counselling, the following need to be discussed:
recurrence risk;
does she want to know whether the fetus is affected?
what options are available (chorionic villus sampling and amniocentesis);
advantages and complications of each of the procedures.

2 Mrs T is a chain smoker who is in her third pregnancy. Her previous babies weighed 2.1 and 2.0 kg at 40 and 39 weeks, respectively. She is now 12 weeks and has come to book under your care. How would you advise her about smoking?
The candidate must cover the following areas:
effect of smoking on fetal size;
smoking and cot death risks;
fetal size and neurodevelopmental disability;
smoking and preterm labour;
smoking and maternal health.

3 Intrauterine fetal death.
Usually this will be in the form of postnatal counselling or pre-pregnancy counselling. The various results must be studied before counselling. Important points to consider during the counselling include the recurrence risk and the plan for the next pregnancy, fetal and maternal monitoring and the timing of the delivery.

4 Counselling about an abnormal screening test.
The questions under prenatal screening could easily be considered as counselling ones. The candidate must be knowledgeable on the various blood tests performed for prenatal diagnosis and their interpretation. The options available for prenatal diagnosis – amniocentesis, chorionic villus sampling and in some cases fetal blood sampling – must be thoroughly understood.

5 Abnormal presentation.
The common ones are breech and transverse lie. The candidate must be aware of the patient's anxiety about associated fetal abnormalities, turning the baby (how, where and when) and the causes of the abnormal lie. Usually most of the women would have had an anomaly scan but it is important even in late pregnancy to do an ultrasound scan to rule out placenta praevia. During the scan, a hydrocephalus must be excluded. During counselling the candidate must, however, not alarm the patient about this possibility!

6 Infections in pregnancy.
This is a wide area but common things occur commonly. Candidates must be aware of the teratogenic effects of chickenpox, *Listeria*, toxoplasmosis and rubella (German measles).

7 Contraception and lactation.
The important points to cover here include the effectiveness of lactation as a form of contraception, the need to avoid the combined oral contraceptive pill if the woman is breast feeding and options such as the progestogen-only pill, implants, barrier methods of contraception and sterilization. If lactational amenorrhoea is to be depended upon, the shortcomings must be highlighted.

ANSWERS

Medical disorders of pregnancy

Question 1
a. Iron-deficiency anaemia.
b. Low haemoglobin.
   Low mean corpuscular volume.
   Low mean corpuscular haemoglobin
      concentration.
c. Breathlessness.
   Easy fatiguability.
   Asymptomatic.
d. Serum ferritin.
e. Parenteral iron.
   Blood transfusion.

Question 2
a. Bossing of the frontal skull.
   Multiple scars on the shins.
b. Sickling test.
   Haemoglobin electrophoresis.
c. Acute sequestration crises.
d. Hourly determination of haemoglobin
      to see if it is dropping.
   Hourly palpation and measurement of
      the splenic enlargement.
e. Liberal and potent analgesics.
   Rehydration.
   Transfusion.

Question 3
a. She may have been transfused.
   There might have been a failure to
      administer anti-D immunoglobulin
      after her previous baby.
   The immunoglobulin administered may
      not have been enough to cover the
      fetomaternal haemorrhage.
   Silent fetomaternal haemorrhages may
      have occurred in the previous or
      index pregnancy without being
      noticed.
b. The baby may be of the same blood
   group as the mother.

There may be ABO incompatibility.
c. Haemolytic anaemia.
   Anaemic heart failure and fetal
      hydrops.
   Intrauterine fetal death.
d. Neonatal jaundice.
   Kernicterus.
e. Intrauterine transfusion.
   Exchange blood transfusion after
      delivery.

Question 4
a. Threatened miscarriage.
   Antepartum haemorrhage.
   Amniocentesis.
   External cephalic version.
   Chorionic villus sampling.
b. Group O rhesus D-negative.
c. Intraperitoneal.
   Intravascular.
d. The fetus (if rhesus positive) will require
   transfusion at an earlier gestation.

Question 5
a. Asymptomatic significant bacteriuria.
b. Symptomatic urinary tract infection.
   This is four times more likely in women
   with untreated symptomatic
   bacteriuria.
c. Urinary tract abnormalities.
   Kidney stones.
   Pylonephritis.
d. Antibiotics with either trimethoprim,
   ampicillin or nitrofurantoin.
e. Ultrasound scan of the kidneys.
   Intravenous urogram 3–4 months after
      delivery.

Question 6
a. Pre-eclampsia (which may occur in
      about 30% of cases).
   Rejection (which may occur in up to
      about 10% of cases).

Premature labour (in about 40–50% of cases).

Intrauterine growth retardation.

Renal impairment (which may occur in up to 15% of patients).

b. Serial full blood counts, blood urea nitrogen (BUN), creatinine, electrolytes; 24-hour creatinine clearance, MSU, plasma proteins and liver function tests.

Serial ultrasound scans for fetal growth.

Blood pressure.

Monitor immunosuppressive drug levels.

c. Caesarean section because of the location of the kidney.

d. Combined oral contraceptive pill. Intrauterine contraceptive device.

Question 7

a. Autoimmune thrombocytopenia.

b. Lupus anticoagulant. Anticardiolipin antibodies. Platelet (IgG) antibody.

c. Serial platelet count.

d. Avoid fetal blood sampling. Ensure platelets are available for transfusion. Avoid traumatic deliveries.

Question 8

a. Systemic lupus erythematosus. Antiphospholipid syndrome.

b. Antiphospholipid antibody. Lupus anticoagulant. Anti-Ro antibodies.

c. Aspirin. Heparin.

d. Serial ultrasound scans. Doppler velocimetry of the uterine artery and umbilical vessels. Biophysical profile. Frequent blood pressure and renal function tests.

Question 9

a. Increased risk of preterm labour by (11–25%).

Increased incidence of neonatal thyrotoxicosis.

Increased incidence of stillbirths (by 8–15%).

b. Identification and quantification of long-acting thyroid stimulating (LATS) hormone.

c. It crosses the placenta and induces transient neonatal thyrotoxicosis.

d. Propranolol (beta-blockers).

e. The baby must be monitored for neonatal thyrotoxicosis for the first six months of life.

Question 10

a. Cardiac disease with slight to moderate limitation of physical activity. Ordinary physical activity causes discomfort.

b. Prematurity. Small for gestational age. Increased maternal mortality.

c. Antibiotic cover in labour should be recommended. Rapidly acting oxytocics should be avoided.

d. To avoid subsequent pregnancies. To be sterilized.

Question 11

a. Intrahepatic cholestasis of pregnancy.

b. Dark urine. Light/pale-coloured stools. Jaundice.

c. Hepatitis viral serology. Ultrasound scan of the hepatobiliary tract. Autoantibodies screen (to exclude primary biliary cirrhosis).

d. Antepartum haemorrhage. Preterm labour. Higher perinatal mortality (due to a higher stillbirth and preterm delivery rate).

e. Monitor liver function tests frequently. Monitor fetal well-being serially. Antipruritics (e.g. cholestyramine) to the mother. Consider vitamin K administration.

Deliver early if pruritus is debilitating or at around 38 weeks.

Question 12
a. Acute fatty liver of pregnancy.
b. Easy fatiguability.
   Malaise.
   Fever.
   Confusion.
c. Maternal mortality.
   Fetal mortality.
   Acute liver failure.
   Renal failure.
   Disseminated intravascular coagulation.
d. Resuscitation.
   Deliver the fetus as soon as possible.
   Monitor to identify any of the complications listed above.
   Haematological back-up is very important.
e. Hyperemesis gravidarum.
   Pre-eclampsia.
   Acute cholestasis of pregnancy.
   Hepatitis.
   Any cause of haemolysis, e.g. malaria, infections, drugs.
   Gall stones/obstruction.

Question 13
a. She should continue taking her antiepileptic medication.
   She should start taking folic acid 0.4 mg daily.
b. Increased incidence of neural tube defects.
c. Her Epilim requirements may increase.
   The baby will need to be screened for congenital anomalies by ultrasound scan.
d. Nausea and vomiting in early pregnancy.
   Increase in blood volume.
   Increase in binding globulins.

Question 14
a. Systemic lupus erythematosus.
b. Miscarriage/early fetal loss.
   Pre-eclampsia.
   Intrauterine growth retardation.

Late fetal loss.
Abruptio placenta.
Fetal heart block.
Neonatal lupus erythematosus.
c. Aspirin.
   Heparin.
d. Serial ultrasound scan.
   Serial Doppler velocimetry.
   Biophysical profilometry.

Question 15
a. Miscarriage.
   Cataract and blindness.
   Congenital heart defects.
   Deafness.
   Mental retardation.
b. Serology – IgG and IgM antibodies.
c. Most cases are asymptomatic.
   Symptoms if present include fever, cough, conjuctivitis, headaches, arthralgia and myalgia.
d. Rubella vaccine with the advice that she should avoid pregnancy for three months.

Question 16
a. Parvovirus B19.
b. May be asymptomatic.
   Arthralgia, fever, malaise, fatigue, depression, sore throat and a rash.
c. Transplacental transfer.
d. Fetal anaemia.
   Hydrops fetalis secondary to anaemic heart failure and manifesting as ascites, pericardial effusion and hepatomegaly.
e. Fetal blood sampling for antibodies and viral studies.

Question 17
a. A DNA virus.
b. Maternal IgG antibody estimation.
c. Cutaneous scarring.
   Limb hypoplasia.
   Missing digits.
   Chorioretinitis, cataracts, hypoplasia of the optic disc.
   Microcephaly.
   Horner's syndrome.

d. Varicella pneumonia.
 Premature labour.
e. The neonate should be given varicella-zoster immunoglobulin.

Question 18
a. A protozoan known as *Toxoplasma gondii*.
b. Most adults are asymptomatic.
 Asymptomatic lymphadenopathy.
 Malaise.
 Sore throat.
 Encephalitis symptoms.
c. Chorioretinitis.
 Microcephaly.
 Hydrocephalus.
 Cerebral calcifications.
 Spontaneous abortions and stillbirths.
 Mental retardation.
 Neonatal jaundice.
d. There is no definitive test to identify infection.
 Demonstration of a rising IgM titre (using paired convalescent samples) is the best method of confirming infection.
e. By administering sulphonamides in combination with pyrimethamine or spiramycin.
f. Avoid raw or poorly cooked meat.
 Wash vegetables properly before eating.
 Careful disposal of cat litters.

Question 19
a. Malaria infection.
b. Blood film for malaria parasites.
c. Drugs to bring down her temperature.
 Antimalarials depending on the recommendations of the School of Tropical Hygiene as there are many strains of chloroquine-resistant malaria.
d. Preterm labour.
 Cerebral malaria which may cause death.
 Severe haemolysis causing anaemia and jaundice.

Question 20
a. Stop the fit with intravenous diazepam.
 Maintain the airway – turning the patient to her side, extending the neck and maybe putting in a Guedel's mouthpiece.
 Prevent the occurrence of subsequent fits by the administration of magnesium sulphate.
b. Eclampsia.
 Epilepsy.
 Meningitis.
 Encephalitis.
 Metabolic disturbance.
 Intracranial tumour.
c. Check her blood pressure.
 Urinalysis.
 Blood sugar.
 Full blood count.
 Urea and electrolytes.
 Liver function test.
d. No. Post fitting, the blood pressure may drop. In addition, some women may fit at lower blood pressures; this obviously depends on the normal blood pressure.
e. Once the woman has been stabilized, deliver the baby vaginally if the cervix is favourable; if not deliver by caesarean section.

Question 21
a. Arrange for her to have a series of blood glucose estimations (fasting, pre- and post-prandial). A glucose tolerance test may be very dangerous as she may in fact be diabetic.
b. Diabetes mellitus.
c. Commence her on insulin.
 Serial blood glucose estimations using BMstix.
 Serial glycosylated haemoglobin or fructosamine.
d. Reduced renal threshold in pregnancy means that a lot of women will have glycosuria in the absence of abnormal glucose metabolism.
e. Nephropathy.
 Retinopathy.

Question 22

a. Glucose tolerance test.
b. Persistent glycosuria.
   Fetal macrosomia.
   Obesity.
   Family history of diabetes mellitus.
   Unexplained stillbirths.
   Polyhydramnios.
   Previous congenital malformations.
c. Ventricular septal defects.
   Coactation of the aorta.
   Sacral agenesis.
   Skeletal abnormalities.
d. It depends on glycaemic control. If poorly controlled, deliver once fetal maturity is achieved. For good control, most units deliver at about 38 weeks' gestation but some allow the women to get to term before delivering.

Question 23

a. Impaired glucose tolerance.
b. Dietary control in the first instance and, if it is unsuccessful, insulin.
c. Fetal macrosomia associated with dystocia.
   Unexplained intrauterine death.
   Polyhydramnios.
d. At 38 weeks' gestation.
e. Stop the insulin and return her to her pre-pregnancy status (without any treatment).
f. She has a higher risk of developing adult-onset diabetes mellitus and therefore will require frequent screening.

Question 24

a. Fetal macrosomia secondary to maternal diabetes.
b. Neonatal hypoglycaemia.
   Neonatal jaundice.
   Neonatal hypocalcaemia.
   Polycythaemia.
   Hypomagnesaemia.
   Respiratory distress syndrome.
c. Glucose tolerance testing for various indications.

d. Obstructed labour.
   Shoulder dystocia.
   Erb's and Klumpke's palsies.

Hypertensive disorders of pregnancy

Question 1

a. Pre-eclampsia.
b. None.
   Headaches.
   Visual disturbances.
   Abdominal pain.
   Nausea and vomiting.
   Confusion and irritability.
c. Full blood count.
   Urea and electrolytes including uric acid levels.
   Liver function test.
   Coagulation profile.
d. Thrombocytopenia.
   Haemolysis.
   Disseminated intravascular coagulation.

Question 2

a. High uric acid levels.
   High creatinine levels.
   Low plasma albumin.
b. Significant proteinuria.
   Raised blood pressure.
   Symptoms of headache, right hypochondrial pain and visual disturbances.
c. Pre-eclampsia.
   Chronic renal disease.
d. Pre-eclampsia occurs for the first time after 20 weeks.
   Renal disease usually predates pregnancy although this may not have been identified before. However, at booking, proteinuria would have been detected.

Question 3

a. Severe pre-eclampsia/fulminating pre-eclampsia.

b. Eclampsia.
   Maternal mortality.
   Renal failure.
   Disseminated intravascular coagulation.
   Cardiovascular accidents such as stroke.
   Haemolysis, elevated liver enzymes and low platelet count (HELLP) syndrome.
   Abruptio placenta.
c. Treat blood pressure with antihypertensives.
   Monitor fetus and deliver if control of blood pressure is difficult.
   Administer steroids to accelerate fetal lung maturity.
   Inform neonatal unit about impending delivery.
   Strict input and output chart.
d. Circulatory overload.
   Disseminated intravascular coagulation.
   Thromboembolism.
   Cardiovascular accidents.

Question 4

a. Primiparity (usually first pregnancies for the father).
   Family history of pre-eclampsia, hypertension and heart attacks.
   Multiple pregnancy.
   Age.
   Systemic diseases such as systemic lupus erythematosus.
b. There are no highly predictive tests but the use of notches at 24 weeks' gestation in the uterine artery Doppler waveforms has been used to identify those at risk of developing pre-eclampsia. Other tests such as the 'Roll-over' test and angiotensin infusion have been used in the USA.
c. There is no definitive means of preventing the disease but the use of low dose aspirin in very high risk groups has reduced the occurrence of very severe disease.

Her blood pressure and urine will need to be monitored very closely.

Question 5

a. Ultrasound for fetal growth and liquor volume.
   Doppler velocimetry of the fetal and umbilical vessels.
b. Blood pressure measurement four times daily.
   Serial (at least twice weekly) full blood counts, urea and electrolytes and uric acid estimation.
   Weekly liver function tests.
   Daily urinalysis for protein and at least once weekly 24-hour urine protein collection.
   Strict input and output chart.
c. Intrauterine growth retardation.
   Intrauterine fetal death.
d. If there is deterioration in the maternal condition, she would be delivered.
   If there is no risk to the mother and the fetus is reasonably healthy, the pregnancy will be prolonged as far as feasible.

Question 6

a. HELLP syndrome.
b. Haemolysis, elevated liver enzymes and low platelet count.
c. Coagulation screen.
   Urinalysis.
d. Deliver the baby as soon as possible.

Question 7

a. Pre-renal renal failure.
b. Inserted a central venous pressure (CVP) line/Swan–Ganz catheter.
   Administer human albumin or colloids.
   Challenge the kidneys with diuretics.
c. Acute tubular necrosis often secondary to poor renal perfusion.
d. Adequately managed, there is usually complete revovery.

Question 8

a. Pre-eclampsia.
b. Intrauterine growth retardation.

c. Check her blood pressure and perform a urinalysis.
d. Arrange hospital admission.
e. Urea and electrolytes.
   Full blood count (specifically looking at the platelets).
   24-hour urinary protein.
   Examination of the retinae (fundoscopy).
   Liver function test.

Antepartum and postpartum haemorrhage

Question 1
a. A woman who has had at least five pregnancies beyond 24 weeks' gestation.
b. Placenta praevia (placenta covering the cervical os).
c. Painless vaginal bleeding.
   Transverse lie of the fetus.
   Unstable lie.
   Breech presentation.
d. Severe maternal haemorrhage.
e. Caesarean section.

Question 2
a. A retroplacental clot.
b. Asymptomatic.
   Abdominal pain with or without vaginal bleeding.
   Symptoms of shock (dizziness and sweating).
c. Pallor.
   Weak and thready pulse.
   Low blood pressure.
   Abdominal tenderness.
   Fundal height bigger than dates.
   Fetal parts difficult to palpate.
   Absent fetal heart sound on auscultation or sonicaid.
d. Disseminated intravascular coagulation.
   Acute renal failure from tubular necrosis.
   Maternal death.

Question 3
a. Syntometrine.
b. For the management of the third stage of labour.
c. With the delivery of the anterior shoulder.
d. Postpartum haemorrhage.
e. Intramuscularly.
   Intravenously.
f. Nausea.
   Vomiting.
   Hypertension.
g. Hypertension.
   Cardiac disease.
   An undelivered second twin.
h. Syntocinon.
   Misoprostol.

Question 4
a. Placenta praevia.
b. Painless bleeding.
   Transverse lie.
   No clinical evidence of concealed haemorrhage.
   No fetal compromise.
c. Placental abruption.
   Unclassified antepartum haemorrhage (APH).
   Placental edge bleed.
   Local cause of the bleeding, e.g. cervical bleeding.
d. Admit into the hospital.
   Intravenous access.
   Full blood count, group and crossmatch.
   Monitor blood loss, maternal and fetal well-being.
e. Ultrasound scan for placental localization.

Question 5
a. Placental abruption.
b. Irritable uterus.
   Tender uterus.
c. Intravenous access.
   Full blood count, group and crossmatch.
   Coagulation profile.

Continuous fetal monitoring.
d. Immediately.
e. If the cervix is favourable, a vaginal delivery should be aimed for; if not, a caesarean section should be performed.

Question 6
a. Missing cotyledon.
b. Asymptomatic.
   Primary postpartum haemorrhage.
   Secondary postpartum haemorrhage.
   Poor uterine involution.
   Endometritis.
c. Intravenous access.
   Group and save.
   Arrange exploration of the uterus and manual removal under general anaesthesia.
d. Cervical lacerations.
   Vaginal tears.
   Perineal tears and episiotomies.
   Ruptured varicose veins.

Question 7
a. Secondary postpartum haemorrhage.
b. Arrange admission into the hospital.
c. Retained products of conception.
   Retained blood clots.
   Infection.
d. Full blood count.
   Group and save serum.
   Ultrasound scan.
e. Antibiotics.
   Evacuation of the uterus.

Question 8
a. Disseminated intravascular coagulation.
b. Low fibrinogen.
   Prolonged clotting time.
   High fibrinogen degradation products.
c. Pre-eclampsia.
   Intrauterine fetal death.
   Amniotic fluid embolism.
   Severe haemorrhage.
   Sepsis.
d. Replacing platelets.
   Infusing fresh frozen plasma.
   Infusion of cryoprecipitate.

Prenatal diagnosis

Question 1
a. This is generally regarded as greater than her age-related risk but the exact figures are uncertain.
b. This is a test done by most units between 14 and 16 weeks' gestation. It measures β-HCG and alpha-fetoprotein and combines this with maternal age to produce a risk.
   The test is only a screening test. It does not accurately identify an affected pregnancy.
c. Chorionic villus sampling.
d. The miscarriage risk is higher 2–4%.
   Higher risk of confined placental mosaicism.
   The test can only be performed at specialized centres.

Question 2
a. The alpha-fetoprotein level is high.
b. Bleeding in pregnancy.
   Wrong dates.
   Multiple pregnancy.
   Missed abortion.
c. Ultrasound scan.
d. Intrauterine growth retardation.
   Unexplained fetal death
   Pre-eclampsia.

Question 3
a. Spina bifida.
b. Raised maternal serum alpha-fetoprotein.
c. Termination.
   Continuation with the pregnancy.
d. To take folic acid before embarking on another pregnancy and continuing with it throughout the first trimester.

Question 4
a. Exomphalos and gastroschisis.
b. In exomphalos, there is a covering membrane.
   In gastroschisis, there is no covering membrane.
c. Karyotyping will be offered in cases of

exomphalos but not to those with gastroschisis. The risk of chromosomal abnormalities is 30–50% in those with exomphalos.

d. Alpha-fetoprotein tends to be raised.

Question 5

a. It shows a raised Down's syndrome risk (1 : 50).

b. Do nothing or have a diagnostic test or amniocentesis (chorionic villus sampling.)

c. Amniocentesis: this involves drawing amniotic fluid; it takes 2–3 weeks for the results to become available; and the miscarriage risk following the test is 0.5–1.0%.

Chorionic villus sampling: this involves taking a sample of the placenta at this stage; the results can be available within 48 hours; and the miscarriage risk following the test is between 2 and 4%.

d. Although there are markers for Down's syndrome, their presence or absence does not necessarily imply an affected or normal fetus. However, the presence of these markers may increase the risk of a fetus being affected.

Question 6

a. One in four.

b. From a chorionic villus sample, provided the particular deletions in the parents have been recognized. It must, however, be emphasized that because there are other deletions which are yet to be identified, no absolute guarantee can be given following a prenatal diagnosis.

c. Polyhydramnios.
Bowel obstruction.
Meconium peritonitis.
Hydrops fetalis.

d. Although most people would perform chorionic villus sampling after 10 weeks' gestation, the test could be performed as early as eight weeks.

Question 7

a. Spina bifida, anencephaly.
Anterior abdominal wall defects (exomphalos and gastroschisis).
Congenital nephrosis.
Teratoma.
Cystic adenomatous malformations of the lungs.

b. Polyhydramnios.
Abnormal lie.
Breech presentation.

c. There is poor swallowing which leads to the accumulation of liquor. In the presence of excessive liquor, the lie of the fetus becomes unstable. In addition, the breech becomes the most dependent part in the absence of a cranial vault.

d. This is thought to be related to the absence of a normal cortisol level in the fetus which appears to play a part in the initiation of labour.

Question 8

a. Alpha-fetoprotein: low level.
β-HCG: high level.

b. It means that her risk of having a baby with Down's syndrome is greater than her age-related risk. It does not mean that her baby has Down's syndrome.

c. If she wishes to find out whether her baby is affected or not, then she would be referred for amniocentesis or chorionic villus sampling (placental biopsy).

d. No test is 100% reliable. However, amniocentesis is very reliable except on the very rare occasion where the maternal cells may be cultured rather than fetal. Placental biopsy (chorionic villus sampling) occasionally may not give an accurate karyotype of the fetus because of confined placental mosaicism.

Question 9

a. After one affected fetus, the risk rises to about 1%.

b. Abnormal nuchal translucency. This is only a screening test.

c. This could be difficult to interpret in multiple pregnancies. In addition, since she has had an affected baby, she would be better off with a definitive diagnosis.
d. Amniocentesis.
e. If one of the babies is affected, it will be difficult to determine which is the affected baby. It would be ethically difficult to offer termination of a normal fetus because the second one is affected.
f. Continue with the pregnancy. Selective fetocide.

Question 10
a. They are likely to be carriers of the sickle cell trait.
b. One in four (25%).
c. Parental haemoglobin electrophoresis.
d. Chorionic villus sampling between 10 and 13 weeks.
e. Miscarriage.
   Fetomaternal haemorrhage leading to rhesus isoimmunization.
   Infection.

Fetal monitoring

Question 1
a. Fetal kick chart (Cardiff 'count-to-ten' chart).
b. When there is a need to monitor the fetus, for example when there are reduced fetal movements, intrauterine growth retardation, hypertension or previous stillbirth.
c. Chose a 12-hour period, preferably between 9 am and 9 pm, and count the number of fetal movements. Once she reaches 10, she should stop and mark the time the 10th movement was felt on the chart.
   Whenever she feels no movements or less than 10 movements within the 12 hours she must contact her midwife, doctor or the hospital.
d. CTG.

Question 2
a. Asymmetrical intrauterine growth retardation.
b. Idiopathic in most cases.
   Hypertension/pre-eclampsia.
   Systemic lupus erythematosus/antiphospholipid syndrome.
c. Fortnightly ultrasound scans for fetal growth and liquor volume.
   Serial Doppler velocimetry of the umbilical artery and middle cerebral arteries.
   Fetal kick chart.
   Weekly CTGs.
   Weekly biophysical profiles.
d. Fetal growth, Doppler scans and CTGs.

Question 3
a. Fetal tachycardia with a fetal heart rate of 175/minute.
   Unprovoked decelerations.
b. Admit onto the labour ward for continuous monitoring.
c. Delivery by caesarean section if the cervix is unfavourable or artificial rupture of the membranes if the cervix is favourable and then start Syntocinon.
d. Ensure that the fetus is monitored continuously and perform a fetal blood sample if this pattern persists.

Question 4
a. A 30-minute CTG.
   Ultrasound scan for liquor volume, fetal tone, gross body movements and breathing.
b. Reduced, absent or reversed end diastolic flow.
c. Fetal kick chart which she herself can keep.
d. Hypoglycaemia.
   Hypothermia.
   Feeding difficulties.
   Necrotizing enterocolitis.
   Infections.
e. Adult hypertensive and cardiovascular diseases.

Neurodevelopmental disabilities.
Diabetes mellitus.
Chronic lung diseases.

Question 5

a. Ultrasound scan for liquor volume.
   Biophysical profile.
   Doppler of the umbilical artery/middle cerebral artery.
   CTG.
   Kick chart.
b. Higher perinatal mortality.
   Meconium aspiration.
   Shoulder dystocia.
   Higher incidence of caesarean section.
c. Length (effacement), position and consistency of the cervix, cervical dilation and station of the presenting part.
d. Ripen the cervix with prostaglandins and then rupture the membranes, followed by Syntocinon if indicated.

Question 6

a. Small for gestational age.
b. Ultrasound scan.
c. Head circumference.
   Abdominal circumference.
   Liquor volume.
d. CTG.
   Doppler of the umbilical artery and middle cerebral artery.
   Biophysical profile.
e. Intrauterine fetal death.
   Fetal distress in labour.
   Oligohydramnios.

Question 7

a. Small for gestational age (intrauterine growth retardation).
b. Ultrasound scan.
c. Head circumference.
   Abdominal circumference.
   Liquor volume.
d. Fetal kick chart.
   CTG.
   Doppler of the umbilical artery.
   Biophysical profile.

e. Intrauterine death.
   Intrapartum fetal acidosis.
   Neonatal hypoglycaemia.
   Long-term morbidity as adults.
   Necrotizing enterocolitis.
   Polycythaemia.
   Hypoglycaemia.

Preterm labour and premature rupture of fetal membranes

Question 1

a. Speculum examination.
   Fern test.
   Nitrazine test.
b. Cord prolapse.
   Preterm labour.
   Intrauterine infection.
c. Twice weekly full blood counts.
   Daily CTG.
   Four-hourly maternal temperature and pulse.
   Daily abdominal palpation.
   Daily inspection of the vulva and pad.
d. Respiratory distress syndrome.
e. Antenatal steroid administration.

Question 2

a. Cervical incompetence.
b. Serial ultrasound scans measuring the length and dilation of the cervix.
c. Cervical cerclage (McDonald or Shirodkar) at 14–16 weeks.
d. Antepartum haemorrhage.
   Established labour.
   Premature rupture of the fetal membranes.
e. Thirty-eight weeks' gestation.

Question 3

a. About 15–25% of women are asymptomatic carriers of beta-haemolytic *Streptococcus* in their genital and gastrointestinal tracts.
b. She should be screened and if the infective organism is isolated, she should be treated.

c. An endocervical swab will be performed and if beta-haemolytic *Streptococcus* is isolated, she should be treated and delivered as well.

d. She should be treated with intravenous antibiotics in labour and the baby should be given prophylactic antibiotics.

e. The baby would have to be observed very closely for any signs of infection.

Question 4

a. Full blood count.
   MSU.
   High vaginal swab (HVS)/endocervical swab.

b. Bacterial vaginosis.
   Beta-haemolytic *Streptococcus*
   Polyhydramnios.
   Congenital uterine malformations.
   Chorioamniotis.
   Any cause of pyrexia.
   Placental abruption.

c. Ritodrine.
   Glyceryl trinitrite.
   Salbutamol.
   Nifedipine.

d. Tachycardia.
   Headaches.
   Tremors.
   Palpitations.
   Sweating and feeling flushed.

e. Pulmonary oedema.

Question 5

a. Preterm labour.

b. Full blood count.
   MSU for MCS.
   High vaginal endocervical swab.

c. Respiratory distress syndrome.
   Intracranial haemorrhage.
   Higher perinatal morbidity and mortality.
   Neurodevelopmental disability.
   Hypothermia.
   Anaemia.
   Infection.
   Neonatal jaundice.

d. Administration of steroids.

e. Ritodrine.
   Salbutamol.
   Glyceryl trinitrite.
   Nifedipine.

Labour (normal and abnormal)

Question 1

a. Failure to progress.

b. Rupture the fetal membranes.

c. Commence Syntocinon.

d. Severe moulding and tight fitting of the fetal head within the pelvis.

e. Emergency caesarean section.

Question 2

a. Ensure that the airway is mantained.
   Intravenous access.
   Intravenous fluids.
   Group and save.

b. Postpartum haemorrhage.
   Amniotic fluid embolism.
   Eclampsia.
   Epilepsy.
   Hypoglycaemia.
   Drug reaction.
   Septicaemia (especially Gram-negative).

c. Haemorrhage.
   Dimple in the fundus.
   Fundus protruding into the vagina.

d. Prompt replacement of the inversion preferably under general anaesthesia.

Question 3

a. Intravenous access.
   Group and crossmatch.
   Intravenous fluid.

b. Rub the uterus to provoke contractions.
   Repeat oxytocins if the uterus is not contracting.
   Examine the placenta to see if it is complete.
   Empty the bladder.

c. Retained placental lobe/cotyledon/membrane.
   Trauma to the cervix, vagina or perineum.
   Coagulation defect.
   Ruptured uterus.

d. Exploration of the uterus under general anaesthesia.

Question 4
a. Ultrasound scan by an experienced operator.
b. Explain the diagnosis to the couple in an empathic way.
   Explain the option, especially the need to preferably deliver vaginally.
   Inform the GP and midwife.
   Explain the need to investigate for the cause of the intrauterine death.
   Give the couple some time alone.
c. Coagulation profile.
   Thyroid function test.
   Glycosylated haemoglobin.
   Kleihauer Betke test.
   Lupus anticoagulant and anticardiolipin antibodies.
   Infection screen (viral, protozoal and bacterial).
d. Examine the fetus.
   Swabs from the nose, throat, ears and mouth.
   Gastric lavage for culture.
   Skin biopsy for karyotype.
   X-rays.
   Autopsy.
e. Histology.
   Culture.
   Cytogenetics.

Question 5
a. She is a grande multiparous woman.
b. Precipitate labour.
   Ruptured uterus.
   Intrapartum haemorrhage.
   Postpartum haemorrhage.
c. Risk of obstructed labour.
   Induction will increase her risk of uterine rupture.
d. Contraceptive advice – possibly sterilization.

Question 6
a. Maternal constant abdominal pain.
   Fetal presented part receding into the abdomen.
   Fetal parts easy to palpate abdominally.
   Bleeding per vaginam.
   Tender abdomen.
b. Laparotomy
c. This will depend on the extent of the rupture. If it is very extensive and will almost invariably lead to rupture in the next pregnancy, then the woman may be better off sterilized. If it is just a s car dehiscence, she should not be sterilized.
d. By elective caesarean section.
e. During pregnancy.

Question 7
a. Cover labour with antibiotics.
b. Administer Syntometrine.
c. Shorten the second stage with a forceps.
d. They increase venous return to the heart and this may result in heart failure.

Multiple pregnancy, polyhydramnios and oligohydramnios

Question 1
a. The number of fetuses present on the scan.
   Whether her dates were correct.
b. Multiple pregnancy.
   Polyhydramnios.
   Pregnancy and other pelvic masses.
   Macrosomic baby.
c. Ultrasound scan.
   Glucose tolerance test.
d. Premature rupture of the fetal membranes.
   Unstable lie.
   Preterm labour.
   Abruptio placenta.
   Cord prolapse.
   Postpartum haemorrhage.

Question 2
a. Twin pregnancy.
b. Exaggerated symptoms of pregnancy.
   Fundal height bigger than dates.

Use of ovulation-induction drugs.
Assisted-conception pregnancy.
c. Hyperemesis gravidarum.
Pre-eclampsia.
Anaemia.
Pressure symptoms (cardiorespiratory compromise, varicose veins of the legs and vulva).
d. Congenital abnormalities.
Polyhydramnios.
Preterm labour.
Placenta praevia.
Abruptio placenta.
Abnormal lie and presentation.
Premature rupture of membranes and preterm labour.

Question 3
a. Retained second twin.
Abruptio placenta after delivery of the first twin.
Locked twins (if the first is breech and the second is cephalic).
b. Primary postpartum haemorrhage due to uterine atony.
c. Intramuscular or intravenous administration of oxytocics with delivery of the anterior shoulder of the second twin.
Oxytocin infusion after delivery of the placenta.
Group and save in labour.
d. The risk of developing ovarian cancer is greater in women who have taken clomiphene citrate for more than 12 months.

Question 4
a. Complete absence of amniotic fluid.
b. Has she drained liquour?
c. Bilateral renal agenesis.
Premature rupture of the fetal membranes.
Obstruction to urinary outflow.
Cystic dysplastic kidneys.
d. Pulmonary hypoplasia.
e. If the anhydramnios is due to renal agenesis, obstruction to outflow or cystic dysplastic kidneys then the

outlook for the baby is very poor. If it is secondary to ruptured membranes and this is of sudden onset, then the prognosis is not too bad.

Question 5
a. Monozygotic twins.
b. The appearance or absence of the lambda sign on an ultrasound scan at around 10–12 weeks will help in the identification of the zygosity of the twins. The presence of a lambda sign will suggest dizygosity while its absence will suggest monozygosity.
c. Twin-to-twin transfusion.
Congenital malformations.
Intrauterine growth retardation.
Polyhydramnios.
d. By ultrasound scan – the donor twin is growth retarded and oligohydramnic, while the recipient twin is larger and may be polyhydramnic.
e. Repeated amniocentesis.
Laser division of the placenta.

Question 6
a. Duodenal atresia.
b. Trisomy 21.
c. Amniocentesis.
Placental biopsy.
Fetal blood sampling.
d. Small bowel obstruction.

Question 7
a. Acute polyhydramnios.
b. Anencephaly.
Duodenal atresia.
Small bowel obstruction.
Spina bifida.
Teratoma (e.g. a sacrococcygeal teratoma).
Haemangioma of the cord or of the fetus.
Cystic fibrosis.
c. Fluid thrill.
d. Therapeutic amniocentesis.
e. The liquor rapidly reaccumulates after tapping.
f. Indomethacin.

g. Fetal renal failure.
   Premature closure of the patient ductus arteriosus leading to pulmonary hypertension.

Question 8

a. Miscarriage (threatened or missed).
   Hyperemesis gravidarum.
   Vanishing triplet syndrome.
b. Iron tablets and folic acid.
c. Preterm labour.
d. Anaemia.
   Hypertension and pre-eclampsia.
   Pressure symptoms.
e. Admission into hospital for bed rest.
   Antenatal steroids to reduce the severity of respiratory distress syndrome in the babies.
f. The most common way is by caesarean section but a vaginal delivery can be possible.

Instrumental delivery

Question 1

a. Neville Barnes's forceps.
b. Maternal exhaustion in the second stage.
   Fetal distress in the second stage.
   At caesarean section.
   Women with cardiac, severe hypertensive or obstructive airway diseases.
c. The cervix must be fully dilated.
   There must be no contraindication to a vaginal delivery.
   The uterus must be contracting.
   The fetal membranes must have ruptured.
   The bladder must be emptied.
   Analgesia must be adequate.
   The fetal position must be occipitoanterior, occipitoposterior or mentoanterior face presentation.
   The operator must have the required skills.
d. Trauma to the genital tract.
   Ruptured uterus.

Facial nerve palsy.
Fractured skull.
Intracranial haemorrhage.

Question 2

a. Silastic ventouse cup.
b. Maternal exhaustion in the second stage.
   Prolonged second stage.
   Abnormal fetal heart rate in the second stage.
   Abnormal fetal heart rate pattern in the late first stage.
c. Cephalohaematoma.
   Laceration of the fetal scalp.
   Neonatal jaundice.
   Chignon.
   Tears of the vagina.
d. When the operator is inexperienced.
   Delivery before full cervical dilation.
e. Extreme prematurity.
   Face presentation.
   Contracted pelvis (contraindications to vaginal delivery).

Question 3

a. Fetal blood sampling in labour.
b. Fetal tachycardia associated with decelerations.
   Fetal bradycardia associated with decelerations.
   Type II or persistent variable decelerations.
   Type I decelerations with meconium-stained liquour.
c. Maternal acidosis.
   Blood mixing with amniotic fluid.
   Fetal and maternal blood mixing.
d. $pH < 7.2$.
   Base excess > -12 mEq/l.
e. Fifteen per cent of normal CTGs are associated with the delivery of acidotic fetuses while 30% of abnormal CTGs are associated with normal fetuses.

Question 4

a. Kielland's forceps:
   Rotation of the fetal head;
   spiral trauma to the maternal tissues;

ruptured uterus;
urinary retention after delivery.
b. Pudendal needle:
for administering pudendal nerve
block before instrumental
deliveries;
haematoma around the pudendal
artery.
c. Fetal scalp electrode:
monitoring of the fetal heart rate;
infection of the scalp.
Laceration of the scalp.

Puerperium

Question 1
a. Breast engorgement and pain.
Abdominal wound pain.
Discharging wound.
Offensive lochia.
Chest pain and cough.
Urinary frequency and dysuria.
Calf pain/swelling.
b. Breasts: engorged, warm and tender.
Chest: crepitations.
Wound: red, warm, indurated and
discharging.
Calf: swollen, warm and tender.
Uterus: tender and poorly involuted.
Vagina: cervix open, offensive lochia.
c. Chest X-ray.
MSU for MCS.
Wound swab.
HVS.
Blood culture.
Ultrasound scan of the calf/venogram.
d. Breast infection.
Wound infection.
Endometritis.
Chest infection.
Urinary tract infection.
Deep venous thrombosis.

Question 2
a. Pulmonary embolism.
b. V-Q scan.

c. Intravenous heparinization.
d. Obesity.
Operative deliveries.
Pre-eclampsia/hypertension.
Family history of deep venous
thrombosis or pulmonary embolism,
prolonged hospitalization or multiple
pregnancy.
e. Protein C and S levels.
Antithrombin III activity.
Lupus anticoagulant/antiphospholipid
syndrome.
Factor V Leiden.

Question 3
a. Postpartum blues.
b. Mood swings.
Insomnia.
Fluctuating appetite.
c. None (there is no recognized biological
cause for puerperal blues).
d. Empathy/understanding.
Support.
Reassurance.
Sedation.
e. Where there is an already existing
marital conflict.

Question 4
a. Postnatal depression (puerperal
psychosis).
b. Insomnia.
Hallucinations.
Delusions.
Feeling of ambivalence towards her
baby.
c. Arrange admission into a mother and
baby psychiatric unit.
d. Tricyclic antidepressants.
e. Thyroid dysfunction.
Toxic reaction to drugs.

Question 5
a. Breast infection.
b. Breast pain.
Engorged breasts.

c. Enlarged, warm and tender breasts.
   Enlarged axillary lymph nodes.
d. Stop breast feeding from the affected
   breast but still express the milk.
   Administer antibiotics.
   Incise and drain if there is an obvious
   abscess.

Question 6

a. Take a swab.
   Commence on antibiotics –
   broad-spectrum and metronidazole.
b. To keep the perineal area dry.
   To have salt sitz baths.
c. To clean the episiotomy site in order to
   get rid of the necrotic tissues.
d. Once the site is clean, healing should
   occur by secondary intention.

Question 7

a. Simple analgesics (e.g. paracetamol)
   and a firm bra.
   Bromocriptine for 10 days.
b. Bromocriptine is an ovulation-
   induction drug and therefore pregnancy
   may result if adequate contraceptive
   advice is not offered.
c. To use a barrier form of contraception.
   Avoid expressing the breast.
d. It may be as short as 3–4 weeks,
   although it may take longer because of
   the emotional problems associated with
   bereavement.

Question 8

a. Sheehan's syndrome.
b. Avascular necrosis of the anterior
   pituitary.
c. Defeminization symptoms: loss of
   pubic and axillary hair, breast and
   vaginal atrophy.
   Hypothyroidism symptoms.
d. Follicle-stimulating hormone.
   Luteinizing hormone.
   Thyroid-stimulating hormone.
   Adrenocorticotrophic hormone.

Serum oestradiol.
e. Replacement therapy.

Abnormal lie and presentation

Question 1

a. Polyhydramnios.
   Placenta praevia.
   Uterine fibroids.
   Ovarian cysts.
   Uterine abormality (e.g. bicornuate
   uterus).
   Idiopathic/unknown.
b. Ultrasound scan.
c. Type of breech presentation.
   Estimated fetal weight.
   Placental site.
d. Cord prolapse.
   Retained after head.
   Breech passing through an incompletely
   dilated cervix.
   Incoordinate uterine contractions.
e. Most obstetricians will perform a
   pelvimetry.

Question 2

a. Unstable lie.
b. Placenta praevia.
c. Premature rupture of the fetal
   membranes.
   Cord prolapse.
d. Admit into hospital.
e. Once placenta praevia has been
   excluded, the lie is likely to become
   stable and if it stays stable for 2–3 days
   she would be allowed home to await
   the onset of spontaneous labour.

Question 3

a. Pain due to red cell degeneration.
   Abnormal presentation.
   Dysfunctional labour.
   Postpartum haemorrhage due to
   subinvolution.
b. Ultrasound scan to exclude a low-lying
   placenta.

c. Elective caesarean section.
d. Conservative management. Unless they are pedunculated subserous fibroids, they must not be removed at caesarean section because of the risk of significant haemorrhage.

Drugs in pregnancy

Question 1
a. Metronidazole 400 mg three times a day for seven days.
b. Nausea and vomiting.
c. Preterm labour.

Question 2
a. Chondrodysplasia punctata.
   Hypoplasia of the nails.
   Microcephaly.
   Optic atrophy.
b. Change her anticoagulation to heparin or low-molecular-weight heparin.
c. Fetal anomaly scan.
d. Until six weeks after delivery.
e. Osteopenia.

Question 3
a. Intramuscular ceftriaxone 250 mg (cephalosporin) or other potent safe antibiotic.
b. Gonococcal ophthalmitis.
c. About four days after delivery.
d. Discharging red eye.
e. Erythromycin eye drops/tetracycline eye drops.
f. Contact tracing and referral to the genitourinary medicine clinic.

Activity stations

Question 1
a. Protein.
b. Urinary tract infection.
   Vaginal discharge.
   Pre-eclampsia.
   Renal disease.
c. MSU.
   Urea and electrolytes.
   Full blood count.
   Blood pressure.

Question 2
a. Nitrites.
b. Urinary tract infection.
c. MSU.
d. Symptomatic urinary tract infection.
   Preterm labour.

Question 3
a. It shows +++ glucose.
b. Random blood glucose.
   Glucose tolerance test.
c. If it is only impaired glucose tolerance, dietary control will be tried first.
   If the test shows frank diabetes mellitus, then she will be commenced on insulin.
d. Fetal macrosomia.
   Unexplained intrauterine fetal death.
   Polyhydramnios.

Question 4
Examine the lower genital tract and take the necessary swabs explaining to the examiner what you would be telling the patient.

Part C
Neonatology

QUESTIONS

1 The chest X-ray shown in Fig. 62 is that of a baby who was delivered at 38 weeks' gestation by emergency lower segment caesarean section because of fetal hypoxia and acidosis. At delivery the infant was noted to be covered in thick meconium. Immediately after delivery the baby developed respiratory distress with increasing tachypnoea, subcostal and intercostal recession, grunting and cyanosis. The chest X-ray was taken at two hours of age.
a. What is the most likely diagnosis?
b. What is the differential diagnosis?
c. What are the most important steps when resuscitating a baby like this?
d. List three complications of this condition.

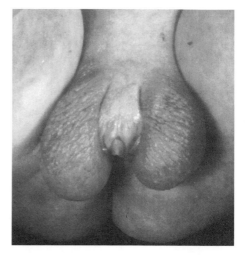

Fig. 63

2 You are called to the delivery suite to see a newborn baby. When you arrive you make a thorough examination of the infant who appears well. The genitalia of this infant are shown in Fig. 63 (see also colour plate section).
a. What information would you give to the parents?
b. List four investigations you would request initially.

3 Figure 64 shows a chart.
a. What is this chart called and what is it used for?
b. What are the external criteria used in this method of assessment?
c. What are the neurological criteria used in this assessment?

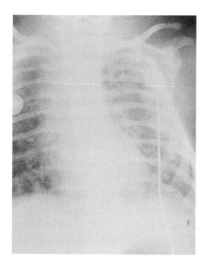

Fig. 62

4 An infant on a postnatal ward collapses at 48 hours of age. The infant was a normal vaginal delivery at term after an uncomplicated pregnancy. Until his collapse he was well. He had breast fed, was reported to have passed meconium at 12 hours of age and had damp nappies. His mother was worried that his urinary stream was poor and not like that of her

External sign	Score 0	1	2	3	4
Oedema	Obvious oedema hands and feet; pitting over tibia	No obvious oedema hands and feet; pitting over tibia	No oedema		
Skin texture	Very thin, gelatinous	Thin and smooth	Smooth: medium thickness. Rash or superficial peeling	Slight thickening. Superficial cracking and peeling especially hands and feet	Thick and parchment-like, superficial or deep cracking
Skin colour (infant not crying)	Dark red	Uniformly pink	Pale pink: variable over body	Pale. Only pink over ears, lips, palms or soles	
Skin opacity (trunk)	Numerous veins and venules clearly seen, especially over abdomen	Veins and tributaries seen	A few large vessels clearly seen over abdomen	A few large vessels seen indistinctly over abdomen	No blood vessels seen
Lanugo (over back)	No lanugo	Abundant: long and thick over whole back	Hair thinning especially over lower back	Large amount of lanugo and bald areas	At least half of back devoid of lanugo
Plantar creases	No skin creases	Faint red marks over anterior half of sole	Definite red marks over more than anterior half: indentations over less than anterior third	Indentations over more than anterior third	Definite deep indentations over more than anterior third
Nipple formation	Nipple barely visible; no areola	Nipple well defined; areola smooth and flat; diameter <0.75 cm	Areola stippled, edge not raised: diameter <0.75 cm	Areola stippled, edge raised: diameter >0.75 cm	
Breast size	No breast tissue; palpable	Breast tissue on one or both sides <0.5 cm diameter	Breast tissue on both sides;one or both 0.5–1.0 cm	Breast tissue on both sides;one or both >1.0 cm	
Ear form	Pinna flat and shapeless. Little or no incurving of edge	Incurving or part of edge of pinna	Partial incurving whole upper pinna	Well-defined incurving whole of upper pinna	
Ear firmness	Pinna soft, easily folded, no recoil	Pinna soft, easily folded, slow recoil	Cartilage to edge of pinna, but soft in places, ready recoil	Pinna firm, cartilage to edge, instant recoil	
Genitalia: Male	Neither testis in scrotum.	At least one testis high in scrotum	At least one testis right down		
Female (with hips half abducted)	Labia majora widely separated, labia minora protruding	Labia majora almost cover labia minora	Labia majora completely cover labia minora		

Neurological sign	Score 0	1	2	3	4	5
Posture						
Square window	90°	60°	45°	30°	0°	
Ankle dorsiflexion	90°	75°	45°	20°	0°	
Arm recoil	180°	90°–180°	<90°			
Leg recoil	180°	90°–180°	<90°			
Popliteal angle	180°	160°	130°	110°	90°	<90°
Heel to ear						
Scarf sign						
Head lag						
Ventral suspension						

Posture: Observed with infant quiet and in supine position. Score **0:** arms and legs extended; **1:** beginning of flexion of hips and knees, arms extended; **2:** stronger flexion of legs, arms extended; **3:** arms slightly flexed, legs flexed and abducted; **4:** full flexion of arms and legs.

Square window: The hand is flexed on the forearm between the thumb and the index finger of the examiner. Enough pressure is applied to get as full a flexion as possible, and the angle between the hypothenar eminence and the ventral aspect of the forearm is measured and graded according to diagram. (Care is taken not to rotate the infant's wrist while doing this manoeuvre).

Ankle dorsiflexion: The foot is dorsiflexed onto the anterior aspect of the leg, with the examiner's thumb on the sole of the foot and other fingers behind the leg. Enough pressure is applied to get as full flexion as possible, and the angle between the dorsum of the foot and the anterior aspect of the leg is measured.

Arm recoil: With the infant in the supine, position the forearms are first flexed for 5 seconds, then fully extended by pulling on the hands, and then released. The sign is fully positive if the arms return briskly to full flexion (score **2**). If the arms return to incomplete flexion or the response is sluggish it is graded as score **1**. If they remain extended or are only followed by random movements the score is **0**.

Leg recoil: With the infant supine, the hips and knees are fully flexed for 5 seconds, then extended by traction of the feet, and released. A maximal response is one of full flexion of the hips and knees (score **2**). A partial flexion scores **1**, and a minimal or no movement scores **0**.

Popliteal angle: With the infant supine and his pelvis flat on the examining couch, the thigh is held in the knee-chest position by the examiner's left index finger and thumb supporting the knee. The leg is then extended by gentle pressure from the examiner's right index finger behind the ankle and the popliteal angle is measured.

Heel to ear manoeuvre: With the baby supine, draw the baby's foot as near to the head as it will go without forcing it. Observe the distance between the foot and the head as well as the degree of extension at the the knee. Note that the knee is left free and may draw down alongside the abdomen.

Scarf sign: With the baby supine, take the infant's hand and try to put it around the neck and as far posteriorly as possible around the opposite shoulder. Assist this manoeuvre by lifting the elbow across the body. See how far the elbow will go across and grade according to illustrations. Score **0:** elbow reaches the opposite axillary line; **1:** elbow between midline and the opposite axillary line; **2:** elbow reaches midline; **3:** elbow will not reach midline.

Head lag: With the baby lying supine, grasp the hands (or the arms if a very small infant) and pull him slowly towards the sitting position. Observe the position of the head in relation to the trunk and grade accordingly. In a small infant the head may initially be supported by one hand. Score **0:** complete lag; **1:** partial head control; **2:** able to maintain head in line with body; **3:** brings head anterior to body.

Ventral suspension: The infant is suspended in the prone position, with examiner's hand under the infant's chest (one hand in a small infant, two in a large infant). Observe the degree of extension of the back and the amount of flexion of the arms and legs. Also note the relation of the head to the trunk. Grade according to diagrams.

If the score for an individual criterion differs on the two sides of the baby, take the mean.

Fig. 64 From Dubowitz L.M.C., Dubowitz V. & Goldberg C. (1970) Clinical assessment of gestational age in the newborn infant. *J. Pediatr.*, **77,** 1–9.

other son. A full septic screen was performed including urine culture. On the neonatal intensive care unit it was noted that the urine output was poor and that urine constantly dribbled from the urethral meatus. The 'bag urine' was reported as: >100 white cells, no red blood cells, >10⁵ mixed coliforms.

a. What is the next investigation you would do in light of the 'bag urine' report.
b. What is the most likely diagnosis?
c. List three other investigations you would perform.

5   A term infant was delivered by elective lower segment caesarean section after an uneventful pregnancy. The APGAR scores were 4 at one minute, 6 at five minutes and 9 at 10 minutes. The baby required resuscitaton with bag and mask ventilation for three minutes and facial oxygen for a further five minutes. By two hours of age the infant was grunting, had a respiratory rate of 90/minute and had marked subcostal and intercostal recession. The temperature was 36 °C and the BMstix was 4. Arterial blood gases taken in air showed: pH 7.10, Pa_{O_2} 5.8 kPa, Pa_{CO_2} 8.6 kPa, HCO_3 15 mmol/l, BE −12.

a. List three diagnoses you would consider.
b. What three investigations would you like to perform?
c. How would you treat this baby?

6   A two-day-old term infant on a postnatal ward has had bilious vomits after every feed since birth. The baby is hungry and feeds well but is yet to pass meconium. Clinical examination reveals a dysmorphic child with a flat occiput, large tongue, low set ears and single palmar creases. A plain abdominal film was taken and is shown in Fig. 65.

a. What does the X-ray show?
b. What condition does this child have?

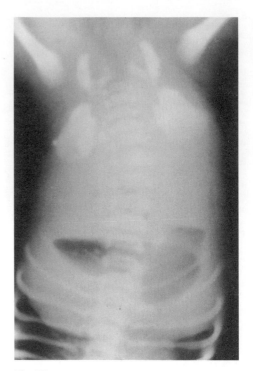

Fig. 65

c. List three further investigations you would perform.

7   A 28-week gestation infant is ventilated for idiopathic respiratory distress syndrome and monitored using an umbilical arterial catheter. The infant is fed with a low birthweight formula from day two but develops abdominal distention and metabolic acidosis on day four. Meconium was passed on day one, but by day four stools contained blood and mucous.

a. What is the most likely diagnosis?
b. What four investigations would you perform?
c. How would you treat this baby?
d. Give one long-term complication of this condition.

8   A full-term infant weighing 3.0 kg is reviewed at four days of age. The midwives are concerned that the baby is lethargic and sleepy, not feeding well and passing watery

stools six times a day. The infant is bottle fed 6–8 hourly with formula feed and takes 25 ml per feed. On day four, the baby's weight is 2.2 kg. Blood was taken for urea and electrolytes and the results are as follows: sodium 158 mmol/l, potassium 4.8 mmol/l, urea 10 mmol/l, creatinine 130 mmol/l.
a. What is the diagnosis?
b. Give two reasons why this has occurred?
c. What investigations would you perform?
d. How would you treat this infant?

9 This infant (Fig. 66, see also colour plate section) was born at 36 weeks' gestation and weighed 4.3 kg.
a. How would you describe this baby's size and appearance?
b. What is the most likely cause for this?
c. List four complications of this condition.

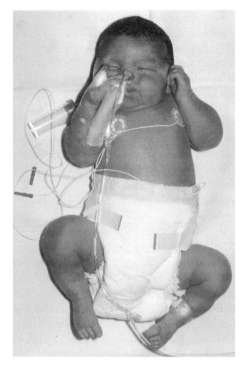

Fig. 66

10 A breast fed infant born at term by difficult ventouse extraction becomes jaundiced at 36 hours of age. On examination the baby appears clinically well other than being markedly jaundiced and having a cephalohaematoma. The serum bilirubin is 350 μmol/l. The baby's mother who is white Caucasian, is blood group O negative and has had one previous live birth (the normal levels of bilirubin are shown in the chart, Fig. 67).
a. Give three possible reasons for this baby's jaundice.
b. What further four investigations would you request in order to identify the cause of this baby's jaundice?
c. How would you treat this baby?

11 Figure 68 (see also colour plate section) shows a baby delivered at term.
a. What abnormalities are shown?
b. What information would you give the parents regarding possible problems in the neonatal period?

c. What information would you give to the parents regarding possible problems in later childhood?

12 During a routine newborn examination you detect a dislocatable hip.
a. What four clinical tests are used to detect dislocated/dislocatable hips?
b. List four important risk factors in congenital dislocation of the hip?
c. What investigation would you order next?

13 Figure 69 shows the weight chart of an infant delivered at 28 weeks' gestation. The baby developed idiopathic respiratory distress syndrome which required ventilation for the first three weeks of life. The baby was then extubated but required 40% head box oxygen until 36 weeks corrected age. Feeding was started on the third day after extubation and by day seven

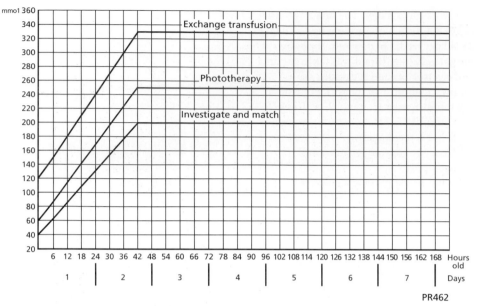

Fig. 67

he was fully nasogastrically fed on breast milk at 175 ml/kg/day.

a. Why is the weight gain poor after 31 weeks' gestation?
b. By what three ways could you improve the weight gain in this baby?

14 Figure 70 shows a card commonly available on most postnatal wards.

a. What test is performed using this card?
b. What three conditions does this test screen for?
c. When should the test be carried out and by whom?
d. Which is the commonest site for sampling for this test?

15 A baby born at 37 weeks' gestation by normal delivery weighs 1.8 kg with a head circumference of 33.5 cm (weight chart shown in Fig. 71). The baby, who required no resuscitation, was put straight to the breast but was unable to feed. At 12 hours of age the baby has still not fed and is

noted to be unwell by midwifery staff. The baby is dressed in a vest and is in a cot with one blanket on the ward nursery where he is being looked after. Paediatric staff ask the midwife to take some baseline observations: peripheral temperature 34.5°C, core temperature 35.5°C, BMstix unrecordable, heart rate 140/minute,

Fig. 68

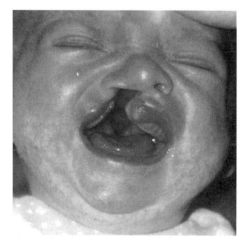

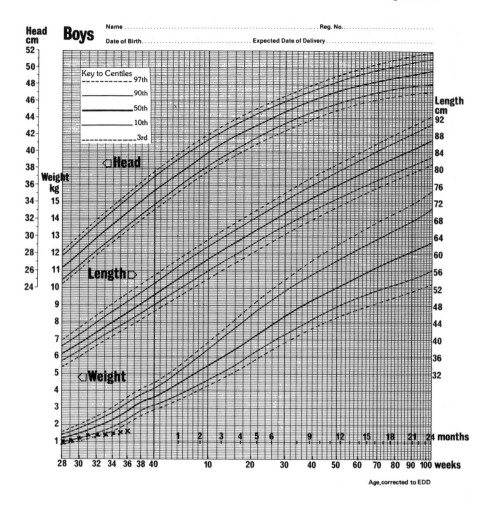

Fig. 69

respiratory rate 70/minute, oxygen saturation 89%.

a. What problem has this baby developed?
b. What factors might have contributed to this baby's condition?
c. What simple measures could have been taken to prevent this?

16 A 26-week gestation infant is delivered vaginally after spontaneous onset of premature labour. The baby makes little spontaneous respiratory effort at birth and is therefore intubated, ventilated and taken to the neonatal unit for further management. An X-ray taken at four hours of age is shown in Fig. 72.

a. What two radiological features are demonstrated?
b. What is the most likely diagnosis?
c. How would you treat this baby's respiratory illness?
d. What antenatal measures affect the course of this disease?

17 The growth chart of a 28-week gestation infant is shown in Fig. 73 along

NEONATAL SCREENING BLOOD TEST
Complete all sections of this form legibly using ball point pen

Surname															

Phenylketonuria

☐ Normal result

☐ Further test required
see comment

First name

Address

Mothers
first name

Birth Wt.				kg	Sex	M ☐		F ☐

Hypothyroidism

☐ Normal result

☐ Further test required
see comment

Please tick if repeat test ☐				District
Date	D	M	Y	Community/Hospital
Birth				
Specimen				GP/Consultant
First Milk Feed				Address of GP or Hospital
Name of Health Visitor or Midwife				

COMMENT

Fill each circle
completely with
ONE DROP of
blood to soak
through to back
of card. Allow to
dry.

HMR 101/6

Fig. 70

with a cerebral ultrasound scan picture
(Fig. 74). An ultrasound scan at 24 weeks'
gestation was normal.
a. What condition does this baby have?
b. Give two reasons for your diagnosis.
c. What is the most likely cause of
this?

18 A five-day-old term baby has collapsed
on the postnatal ward. The baby was well
at birth and fed well for the first three days
of life; however, over the last 48 hours he
has been reluctant to feed and has become
sweaty although not pyrexial. Examination
reveals a deeply cyanosed baby in extremis.
The baby is tachycardic with a heart rate of
200/minute. Brachial pulses are weak but
palpable, but femoral pulses are absent. On
auscultation there is a gallop rhythm,
normal heart sounds and no murmurs. The
respiratory rate is 60/minute with marked
respiratory distress. The baby has
hepatomegaly 4 cm below the costal
margin. A chest X-ray shows cardiomegaly
with plethoric lung fields.
a. What is the most likely diagnosis?

b. What is the main reason for this
diagnosis?
c. What four investigations would you
like to perform?
d. How would you treat this baby?

19 A term baby aged two days is about to
go home when it is noticed that he has not
yet passed meconium. The baby is well,
examination is normal, the anus is
normally placed and per rectum
examination resulted in an explosive bowel
action. A contrast enema was performed
and the film shown in Fig. 75 was
obtained.
a. What does the contrast study show?
b. List two possible diagnoses.
c. What two further investigations would
you like to perform?
d. What further treatment may you offer?

20 Part of the newborn examination
includes detection of the red reflex.
a. How would you detect a red reflex in a
neonate?
b. Give two causes of absent red reflex in a
neonate.
c. What three maternal conditions may
predispose to the absence of this reflex?

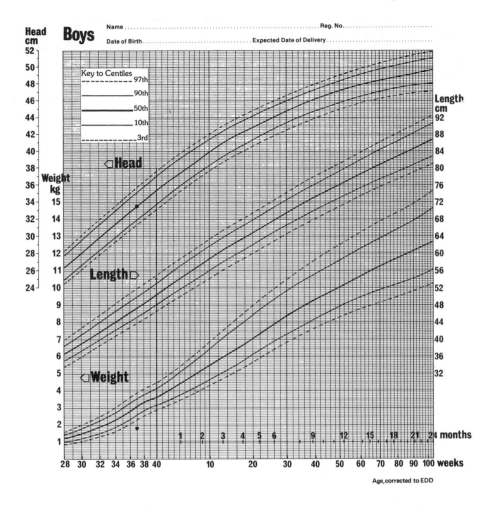

Fig. 71

21 A baby was deliverd at 36 weeks' gestation by emergency lower segment caesarean section because of fetal distress. The only complicating factor was polyhydramnios throughout the pregnancy. The baby was in good condition at birth and required no resuscitation. At six hours of age the nursery nurse became worried because the baby was producing copious amounts of saliva and became dusky during attempts to bottle feed.

a. What is the most likely diagnosis?
b. Name four other known associated features.
c. What investigation(s) would you carry out?
d. How would you treat this baby initially?

22 This ECG (Fig. 76) was taken from a baby at 18 hours of age. The baby was born vaginally at term after an apparently uncomplicated labour. The ECG was ordered after the baby was thought to have a slow heart rate at the newborn examination. There was no maternal

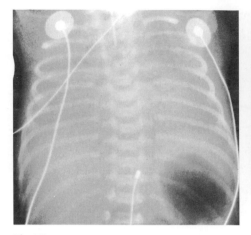

Fig. 72

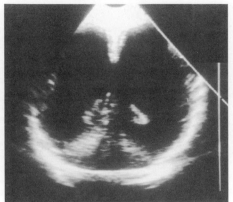

Fig. 74

Fig. 73

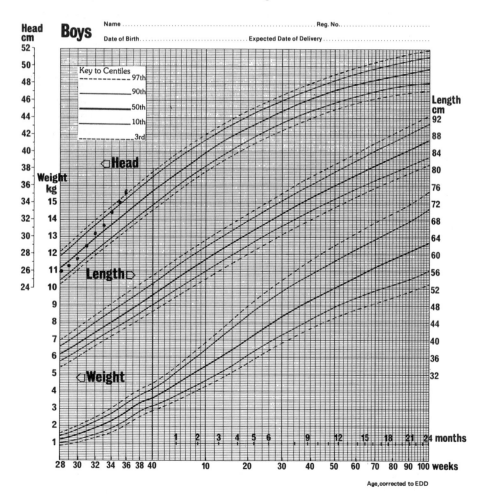

Head
cm

Boys

Name ....   Reg. No. ....

Date of Birth .... Expected Date of Delivery ....

Length
cm

Age, corrected to EDD

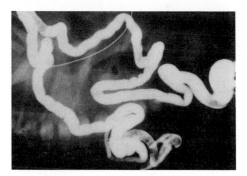

Fig. 75

illness of note but the neonatal Senior House Officer noticed that the mother had a rather odd facial rash.

a. What does this ECG show?
b. What is the significance of the facial rash in the mother?
c. What three maternal investigations might you perform?
d. What other three obstetric complications may be associated with this condition?

23 An infant delivered at 34 weeks' gestation became unwell at two weeks of age. Up until this time he had been cared

for on a neonatal unit, and required tube feeds only. He then began to be less interested in feeds, was rather sleepy, developed bicycling movements of his limbs and jerking movements of his eyes. This baby's mother is well and is on no medication. There is a family history of epilepsy.

a. What investigations would you perform?
b. How would you treat this baby?
c. What is the diagnosis?
d. What is the most likely cause of this condition?

24 This baby (Fig. 77, see also colour plate section) was born after a pregnancy

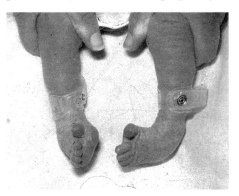

Fig. 76   **Fig. 77**

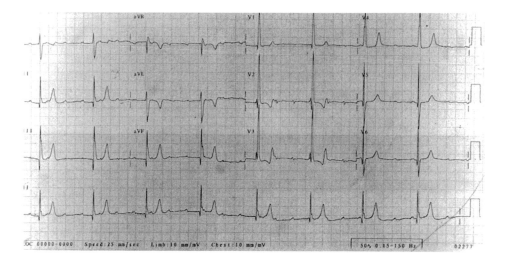

that was complicated by oligohydramnios.

a. What abnormality does this show?
b. What other two anomalies should be actively sought?
c. How is this condition treated?

25 All babies have a Guthrie test taken in the first few days of life. This test is taken from a heel-prick capillary blood sample. This technique is also widely employed on neonatal units.

a. List in order the five steps you would take to obtain a heel-prick sample.
b. Which part of the heel would you take blood from?

ANSWERS

Question 1

a. Meconium aspiration syndrome (MAS).
b. Neonatal pneumonia.
c. Suction of the airways.
   Laryngoscopic sucking and inspection of the cords.
   Endotracheal suction of the meconium seen below the cords.
d. Pneumothorax.
   Persistent pulmonary hypertension.
   Hypoxic ischaemic encephalopathy (including convulsions).
   Renal failure.
   Syndrome of inappropriate antidiuretic hormone secretion (SIADH).
   Hypotension and secondary infection.

COMMENTARY

a,b. The most likely diagnosis is MAS. The chest X-ray shown is characteristic of MAS with widespread patchy infiltration and hyperinflation throughout both lung fields. In addition there is a history of fetal hypoxia and acidosis and meconium-stained liquor which therefore makes MAS likely. The differential diagnosis should include neonatal pneumonia which cannot be excluded from the X-ray appearances.

Wrong answers:
(i) Transient tachypnoea of the newborn (TTN). Although this condition affects term infants and is more common after lower segment caesarean section, the chest X-ray shown here is not compatible with TTN. In TTN X-ray changes include hyperinflation, perihilar streaking, prominent perihilar vascular markings and fluid in the interlobar fissures.
(ii) Idiopathic respiratory distress syndrome (IRDS). This is a condition affecting primarily preterm infants and is

caused by lung immaturity and surfactant deficiency. Affected infants have marked respiratory distress and a characteristic chest X-ray appearance showing fine granular opacification of the lung fields with an air bronchogram, where air-filled bronchi stand out against the atelectatic lungs.

c. MAS occurs when an infant inhales meconium as it takes its first breaths after delivery. The most important part of the management of these infants is in the removal of as much meconium as possible from the airway immediately after delivery. In infants delivered vaginally the mouth and nose should be gently sucked out as soon as the head has crowned. In infants delivered by caesarean section the mouth and nose should be gently sucked out as soon as the head is delivered. In addition, it is important that all infants have their airways cleared of meconium under direct vision and that the vocal cords are inspected where the meconium is thick. If meconium is seen below the cords then direct endotracheal suction is required. This may need to be repeated several times until the suction catheters are clear of meconium.

Wrong answers:
(i) Bag and mask or endotracheal ventilation. This should not be started under any circumstances until the airway has been cleared of meconium. Vigorous bagging will only serve to disperse meconium to the lung peripheries.
(ii) Bronchial lavage. This is not recommended as it is damaging to lung tissue, removes surfactant and has not been shown to be of benefit in the development of MAS.

(iii) Clamping of the chest wall. This in theory prevents the infant from taking a breath until the cords have been visualized and therefore prevents inhalation of meconium. This rather barbaric practice has never been shown to prevent MAS and should not be attempted.

c. The commonest complications include: pneumothorax, persistent pulmonary hypertension, hypoxic ischaemic encephalopathy (including convulsions), renal failure, SIADH, hypotension and secondary infection.

Question 2
a. Genitalia are ambiguous.
   Child needs investigating before gender can be assigned.
   Once gender is determined, treatment will be planned and life should be normal.
b. Karyotype.
   17-hydroxyprogesterone (17-OHP).
   Serum and urinary urea and electrolytes.
   Blood pressure.
   Serum glucose.
   Abdominal ultrasound.

COMMENTARY
a. This infant has ambiguous external genitalia. When discussing this with parents one should never guess the sex of the child. The parents should be told that the infant has genital abnormalities which need to be investigated fully and that until such time as the results of the investigations are known no gender should be ascribed to the child. The parents should understand that the cause can be determined and that the appropriate sex for rearing the child and treatment can be planned. Parents should also be aware that there is no reason why the child should not lead a full and healthy life but that fertility cannot be guaranteed.

b. Initial investigations should include the

following:
(i) Karyotype: provides the genetic sex of the infant.
(ii) 17-OHP: the commonest cause of ambiguous genitalia is congenital adrenal hyperplasia. Five specific enzyme defects are recognized for this condition, the commonest being 21-(alpha) hydroxylase deficiency and 11-(beta) hydroxylase deficiency. The key metabolite for the diagnosis of 21-(alpha) hydroxylase deficiency is 17-OHP, which is elevated and can be measured in blood or urine. The key metabolite in diagnosing 11-(beta) hydroxylase deficiency is 11-deoxycortisol, which is elevated. These tests should be carried out after three days of age as prior to this, results are equivocal as they will reflect maternal levels.
(iii) Serum and urinary electrolytes: some forms of congenital adrenal hyperplasia cause salt-losing states. Here the block in adrenocortical steroid synthesis is at the 21-hydroxylase step which affects aldosterone as well as cortisol pathways. Inadequate production of aldosterone results in renal salt loss and affected infants can become seriously ill from salt depletion and may present in Addisonian crisis. Characteristically one finds hyponatraemia, hyperkalaemia and acidosis.
(iv) Blood pressure: salt wasters may be hypotensive whereas those infants with 11-(alpha) hydroxylase deficiency will eventually become hypertensive.
(v) Serum glucose: hypoglycaemia can occur particularly in adrenocortical insufficiency causing an Addisonian crisis.
(vi) Abdominal ultrasound: this is primarily used to look for gonads. Alternatively a contrast study of the genital orifice is a useful way of outlining genital anatomy.

Question 3
a. Dubowitz chart used for the assessment of neonatal gestational age.

b. Presence of lanugo hair.
   Plantar skin creases.
   Nipple and genital formation.
c. Posture, square window, arm and leg recoil, ankle dorsiflexion, poplited angle, head to ear, scarf sign, head lay and ventral suspension.

Question 4
a. Suprapubic aspiration of the bladder.
b. Urinary tract infection.
c. Serial urea and electrolytes.
   Serial blood pressure measurements.
   Abdominal ultrasound scan.
   Micturating cystourethrogram (MCUG).
   Diethylenetriamine penta-acetic acid (DTPA).

COMMENTARY
a. A suprapubic aspiration of the bladder is mandatory in diagnosing urinary tract infections in neonates. The 'bag urine' report here shows a mixed growth which may be due to contamination of the skin with faeces. The only way to obtain a clean urine specimen in neonates is by suprapubic aspiration which should be performed as a first line investigation in a collapsed neonate. Clean catch specimens are acceptable in older infants but are difficult to collect in the neonate and have no place if the child is ill.

b. This infant is septiceamic from a urinary tract infection which is most likely to be secondary to posterior urethral valves. Most infants with urinary tract infections have an associated septicaemia, although in some the diagnosis is only made on routine testing for prolonged jaundice. A history of poor urinary output and poor stream in a male infant needs urgent investigation to exclude posterior urethral valves. The majority of infants with urethral valves are diagnosed only after they have become ill with a urinary tract infection.

c. Further investigation of the renal tract is essential as up to 50% of infants with a urinary tract infection will have an underlying abnormality. Any infant suspected of having posterior urethral valves with urinary tract infection should undergo all of the following tests initially:
(i) Serial urea and electrolytes and creatinine measurements.
(ii) Serial blood pressure measurements.
(iii) Abdominal ultrasound scan: this will assess gross anatomy, e.g. hydronephrosis or distended bladder.
(iv) MCUG: this is used to detect anomalies of the bladder, the bladder neck and the uretha, and will detect vesicoureteric reflux which can cause renal scarring if severe.
(v) DTPA scan: this will assess renal function, but is only useful after about three months of age.

Question 5
a. Infection with group β-haemolytic *Streptococcus*.
   Neonatal pneumonia – bacterial or viral.
   Pneumothorax.
   Pulmonary hypoplasia.
   Persistent pulmonary hypertension of the newborn.
   Congenital malformation, e.g. diaphragmatic hernia, cystic lung, etc.
   Congenital heart disease.
   Transient tachypnoea of the newborn.
b. Chest X-ray.
   Blood culture.
   Full blood count including differential white cell count.
   ECG.
   Echocardiogram.
   C-reactive protein.
c. Intubation.
   Ventilation.
   Sedation.
   Treat metabolic acidosis with bicarbonate, Tris (hydroxymethyl) aminoethane or plasma.

COMMENTARY

a. The differential diagnoses of respiratory distress in a term infant are varied and include extrapulmonary conditions. The diagnosis can usually be confirmed, or other diagnoses excluded, after taking a history, performing a clinical examination and taking a chest X-ray. Neonatal pneumonia and infection with group β-haemolytic *Streptococcus* can often mimic and coexist with other conditions and therefore all infants with respiratory distress should be covered with antibiotics. Congenital anomalies will usually be confirmed by a chest X-ray, including congenital heart disease which if presenting early will have either cardiomegaly, oligaemia or hyperaemia of the lung fields.

Wrong answers:
(i) Respiratory distress syndrome. This condition usually affects premature infants and rarely affects term infants.
(ii) Metabolic disease. Although this can cause metabolic acidosis and tachypnoea, it does not usually cause repiratory acidosis and CO_2 retention.
(iii) Bronchopulmonary dysplasia. This is chronic lung disease of prematurity.

b. A chest X-ray is clearly essential in all cases. Other investigations should include: blood culture, full blood count including differential white count, ECG, echocardiogram and C-reactive protein.

c. Unless there is a pulmonary air leak or congenital heart disease this infant needs intubation, ventilation and sedation. If an air leak is present the child should have this drained and be given oxygen via a head box. If the child has cyanotic congenital heart disease then ventilation may still be required particularly if prostaglandins are to be given. The blood gases show profound mixed metabolic and respiratory acidosis, with evidence of poor oxygenation. The only treatment option in the absence of an air leak is mechanical ventilation. After intubation the blood gases need to be repeated as the infant may still have a metabolic component to the acidosis which should be treated with bicarbonate, THAM or plasma. As infection cannot be excluded antibiotics should be given to all infants with respiratory distress after blood cultures have been taken.

Wrong answers:
(i) Head box oxygen. Given the blood gases there is no place for this.
(ii) Continuous positive airway pressure ventilation. Again given the blood gases and clinical condition one should not use this but go directly to intubation and ventilation.

Question 6
a. Double bubble appearance in the abdomen.
b. Down's syndrome.
c. Karyotype.
Upper gastrointestinal (GI) contrast study.
Echocardiogram.
Lower GI contrast study.
Rectal biopsies.

COMMENTARY
The X-ray shows the classic double bubble found in duodenal atresia. The child has Down's syndrome. The diagnosis will need to be confirmed by performing a karyotype. However, other investigations which must be considered include: upper GI contrast study, echocardiogram (congenital heart disease should be actively looked for in Down's syndrome babies) and lower GI contrast study (in this baby there had been no passage of meconium by 48 hours). A further gut atresia and Hirschprung's disease need to be excluded by rectal biopsies.

Question 7

a. Necrotizing enterocolitis (NEC).
b. Plain abdominal X-ray.
   Clotting screen.
   C-reactive protein.
   Blood gases.
   Full blood count.
c. Nil by mouth.
   Triple antibiotic therapy (penicillin, gentamicin and metronidazole).
   Parenteral nutrition via long line.
   Correct metabolic acidosis.
   Treat hypotension with inotropes.
   Surgery in severe cases.
d. Bowel stricture.

COMMENTARY

a. NEC is an acquired condition affecting predominantly preterm infants. The cause is unknown but predisposing factors include: asphyxia, hypoxia, feeding with hyperosmolar feeds and conditions of poor gut perfusion, e.g. hypotensive states or where umbilical lines are present. NEC is characterized by inflammation, ulceration and sometimes perforation of the bowel. Mucosal injury allows secondary infection with gas-producing organisms which cause the characteristic radiographic appearances of pneumatosis intestinalis.

b. All infants with suspected NEC should have a series of plain abdominal X-rays taken. A lateral 'shoot through' film may be required if perforation is suspected. In addition blood cultures, full blood count including differential white count, clotting screen, C-reactive protein and arterial blood gases should be taken.

c. If NEC is suspected the infant should be kept nil by mouth to rest the gut and be treated with triple antibiotic therapy of penicillin, gentamicin and metronidazole, depending on individual practice. In addition, nutrition shoud be provided parenterally via a long line and all umbilical lines should be removed.

Metabolic acidosis and disseminated intravascular coagulation are common and should be corrected according to local unit policy. Hypotension should be treated with inotropic support and analgesia provided with opiates. A paediatric surgical opinion should be sought as surgery is required in the most severe cases.

d. Strictures occur in about 15% of infants. Lactose intolerance occurs in 5–10% of infants and a recurrence of NEC in about 5%. Those infants who undergo surgery and undergo gut resection are prone to diarrhoea and short gut syndrome depending on the amount of gut resected.

Question 8

a. Hypernatraemic dehydration.
b. Inadequate feeding (frequency and volume).
   Diarrhoea.
c. Serial serum urea and electrolytes.
   Urinary urea and electrolytes.
   Packed cell volume.
   Stool microscopy and culture.
   Stool chromatography.
   Blood gas analysis.
   Blood pressure.
d. Intravenous fluids as 10% dextrose.

COMMENTARY

Hypernatraemic dehydration has occurred because: (i) the baby has been given inadequate amounts of milk feed, and (ii) the baby has diarrhoea. By the fourth day most infants will take 100–120 ml/kg/day given as a four-hourly bottle. This baby should therefore take 300–360 ml/day which is equivalent to 50–60 ml/bottle every four hours. A newborn baby should not be left for more than four hours without a feed as they are liable to become hypoglycaemic. In this case both the time interval between feeds and the volume given are inadequate, causing this baby becoming severely dehydrated. In addition the baby has diarrhoea which increases the dehydration. This infant has undergone dramatic weight loss which is also an indicator of dehydration. Newborn infants and particularly premature infants are prone to hypernatraemic dehydration if their intake of fluid is inadequate or if there are excessive fluid losses, e.g. from vomiting, diarrhoea, phototherapy units or overhead heaters.

The main problem here is dehydration, i.e. water loss, not sodium overload. Hypernatraemia is assocated with high serum osmolality and therefore the serum sodium should be reduced slowly to avoid convulsions. Intravenous fluids should be given as 10% dextrose only until the serum sodium is within the normal range when oral feeding can be reintroduced.

Question 9

a. Macrosomic.
b. Poorly controlled maternal diabetes mellitus.
c. Hypoglycaemia.
   Idiopathic respiratory distress syndrome.
   Congenital heart disease.
   Cardiomyopathy.
   Polycythaemia.
   Sacral agenesis.
   Shoulder dystocia.

COMMENTARY
This baby is large for gestational age, the weight being over the 97th centile. The appearance is described as macrosomic. The most likely cause for this appearance is maternal diabetes. The complications are numerous and varied and include: hypoglycaemia, idiopathic respiratory distress syndrome, congenital heart disease, cardiomyopathy, polycythaemia, sacral agenesis and shoulder dystocia.

Question 10

a. Rhesus incompatibility.
   ABO incompatibility.
   Cephalohaematoma.

b. Full blood count.
   Packed cell volume and blood film.
   Blood group and Coombs' test.
   Clotting screen.
   Split bilirubin.
   Urea and electrolytes.
   Liver function test.
c. Phototherapy.
   Regular bilirubin checks.
   Adequate hydration via breast feeding, nasogastric tube feeding or intravenous fluids.

COMMENTARY
a. The possible causes for this infant's jaundice include rhesus incompatibility as the mother is rhesus-negative. Other causes include ABO incompatibility, other haemolytic disorders, dehydration and as a consequence of the cephalohaematoma.

Wrong answers:
(i) Physiological jaundice. This is common in term infants but reaches its peak at about four days. This baby has a very high bilirubin level at less than 48 hours which by definition cannot be physiological.
(ii) Breast milk jaundice. This does not appear in the first few days of life, rarely causes bilirubin levels of this magnitude and should be a diagnosis of exclusion.
(iii) Neonatal hepatitis and multiple causes of prolonged jaundice. These occur later and may have a significant conjugated element to the jaundice.

b. A full blood count, packed cell volume and blood film are mandatory, as are blood group and Coombs' test. A clotting screen and split bilirubin would be helpful. Urea and electrolytes should be considered if dehydration is likely, but only after the previous tests.

c. The baby should receive phototherapy and have regular bilirubin readings as well as repeat full blood counts. The baby should have adequate breast milk feeds with additional fluid given as water if necessary. If the baby is dehydrated or too sleepy to breast feed, fluids should be given by nasogastric tube or intravenously.

Question 11

a. Unilateral cleft lip and palate.
b. Explain the condition to the parents and warn them that infants often look unattractive.
   A major problem is that of feeding although special teats are available.
   Regurgitation and repeated chest infections may be common.
c. Cosmetic results are very good.
   Show the parents photographs of treated children (before and after surgery).
   There are often problems with speech but a speech therapist will help.
   Middle ear infections are common.
   Dentition is often delayed.

COMMENTARY

The baby has a unilateral cleft lip and palate. A cleft lip with or without cleft palate occurs in about 1 : 1000 births. These defects occur together in about 70% of cases and may be unilateral, bilateral or midline. Midline clefts are rare and are associated with severe cerebral anomalies, e.g. holoprosencephaly. Clefts of the palate can affect the hard palate, the soft palate or both. Parents need a full explanation of this condition at birth. The infants look unattractive and the parents should be shown before and after photographs.

Problems in the neonatal period are few and usually related to feeding. It is possible to breast feed but feeding is difficult. A variety of special teats are availabe to help feeding babies with a cleft palate and it often takes a while to find a teat that suits a particular baby. Regurgitation down the nose and recurrent episodes of aspiration can be a problem. If the cleft is severe an orthodontic plate may be required to help bring the gum margins together.

The cosmetic result of cleft repairs is very good, although many of these children go on to have problems throughout childhood. There are often problems with speech and a speech therapist should always be involved. In addition middle ear infections are common due to Eustachian tube dysfunction. Hearing needs regular assessment. Dentition is often delayed and there may be malocclusion.

Question 12

a. Unequal leg length.
   Asymmetry of skin creases on the thigh.
   Ortolani's sign.
   Barlow's (dislocation) test.
b. Breech presentation.
   Family history.
   Sex.
   Multiple congenital abnormalities.
c. Ultrasound scan of both hips.

COMMENTARY

Clinical screening for congenital dislocation of the hip should include observation of the infant looking for unequal leg length and asymmetry of skin creases on the thigh. Other tests include Ortolani's (reduction) test and Barlow's (dislocation) test. Important risk factors in congenital dislocation of the hip are presentation (breech vs vertex ratio 10 : 1), family history (the inheritance is polygenic and recurs in families at a rate of around 1 : 30), sex (female : male ratio 6 : 1) and multiple congenital abnormalities particularly those concerned with the musculoskeletal system, e.g. arthrogryposis, spina bifida, etc. The next investigation should be an ultrasound scan of both hips by an experienced ultrasonographer. There is no place for a plain X-ray of the hips at this stage as the femoral epiphyses are not ossified.

Question 13

a. Inadequate caloric intake after extubation.

b. Respiratory support will reduce energy necessary for breathing.
Increase volume of feeds.
Caloric supplement.

COMMENTARY

a. This baby was mechanically ventilated until three weeks of age (31 weeks corrected age). During this time he was fed 175 ml/kg/day of breast milk. Whilst ventilated the energy required for breathing would have been small and therefore the calorie content of the breast milk would have been sufficient to allow weight gain. At three weeks of age the baby was extubated into head box oxygen. His work of breathing then increased dramatically now that he was no longer being given respiratory support. His caloric requirement therefore also increased. Clearly the calorie content of the breast milk is no longer sufficient for this baby and he is failing to gain weight.

b. There are several options available to improve the weight gain in this baby:
(i) As this baby has a high relative oxygen requirement and has increased work of breathing, he may benefit from respiratory support in the form of nasal continuous positive airway pressure. This would decrease his work of breathing and may allow him to grow.
(ii) The volume of the feeds may be increased to 200 ml/kg/day. This should be carried out with caution in premature infants fed nasogastrically who have respiratory distress as they are prone to gastro-oesophageal reflux and may aspirate.
(iii) A calorie supplement or breast milk fortifier could be added to the breast milk. This would provide increased calories in the same volume of milk.

Question 14

a. Guthrie test.

b. Phenyketonuria.
Congenital hypothyroidism.
Cystic fibrosis.

c. After two days of life.
By a midwife in the hospital or community.

d. Heel.

COMMENTARY

The Guthrie test screens for phenyketonuria, congenital hypothyroidism and cystic fibrosis. It is usually taken after the first two days of life as the screening test for phenyketonuria requires the infant to have been on milk feeds for 48 hours. The timing of the test generally means that it is taken by a midwife either in hospital or the community. In the case of premature or ill babies the Guthrie test may be delayed until milk feeds have commenced and in this case may be taken on the neonatal unit.

Question 15

a. Hypothermia.

b. Asymmetrical growth retardation.
Inadequate dressing.
Nursed in a room with open windows.
Baby was put straight to the breast after delivery.

c. Dry and wrap in warm towels after delivery.
Nursed in warm room free of draught.
Use heat shields, overhead heaters or heat mattresses.

COMMENTARY

b. This baby has become hypothermic and his subsequent symptoms are as a result of this. There are a number of reasons why this baby has become hypothermic:
(i) This baby is asymmetrically growth retarded, and will have great difficulty in maintaining his body temperature as he will have little subcutaneous fat, little in

the way of brown fat and glycogen stores and a limited ability to shiver.

(ii) The baby was put straight to the breast after delivery and unless he was dried and well wrapped he would be at risk of cold stress secondary to heat loss by evaporation.

(iii) The baby was inadequately dressed even for the summer months.

(iv) The baby was nursed in a room with an open window and would be at risk of heat loss by convection or radiation.

Newborns attempt to conserve heat when exposed to cold stress by the following means:

(i) Peripheral vasoconstriction.

(ii) Increased heat production by increased metabolism and oxygen consumption and by shivering.

(iii) Non-shivering thermogenesis using brown fat stores.

This baby has clearly made attempts to conserve heat but as he is small for dates these means are likely to be ineffective for the reasons given above. He has therefore become cold, peripherally shut down, hypoglycaemic as all glycogen stores have been used and tachypnoeic and hypoxic secondary to increased oxygen consumption.

c. A number of very simple measures can prevent hypothermia and its subsequent problems:

(i) At delivery babies should be dried and wrapped in warm towels, thus preventing heat loss by evaporation and conduction.

(ii) To prevent heat loss by radiation and convection babies should be adequately dressed and wrapped even in warm weather.

(iii) Nurseries should be warm and free from draught even in summertime.

(iv) Heat shields, overhead heaters, heated mattresses or incubators can all help to minimize heat loss in small but otherwise well infants.

Question 16

a. Bilateral air bronchograms.
Dense reticular pattern throughout both lung fields (the so-called 'solid' appearance).

b. Idiopathic respiratory distress syndrome (IRDS).

c. Respiratory support in the form of mechanical ventilation with oxygen. Administer exogenous surfactant. Intravenous antibiotics to cover infections.

d. Steroids such as dexamethasone.

COMMENTARY

The X-ray shows bilateral air bronchograms and a dense reticular pattern throughout both lung fields giving the lungs a rather 'solid' appearance. The most likely diagnosis is IRDS or hyaline membrane. It is important to note, however, that these cannot be distinguished from infection on clinical or radiological grounds. As this infant is premature IRDS is the most likely diagnosis. As this baby made poor respiratory effort at birth he requires effective respiratory support in the form of mechanical ventilation with oxygen. The baby should be kept well oxygenated ensuring that the Po_2 is kept within the normal range. Exogenous surfactant should be given via the endotracheal tube as soon as possible and antibiotics should be given to cover infection. The widespread use of dexamethasone antenatally has substantially altered the natural history of IRDS.

Question 17

a. Hydrocephalus.

b. Large head circumference.
Fluid space within the skull.

c. Intraventricular haemorrhage.

COMMENTARY

This baby has hydrocephalus. The growth chart shows a progressive increase in head size which crosses the centile lines indicating accelerated head growth. The ultrasound scan shows massive dilation of the lateral ventricles and little surrounding brain tissue. In a premature infant the most likely cause of hydrocephalus is secondary to intraventricular haemorrhage. Post-haemorrhagic hydrocephalus is communicating in 85% of cases as a result of the arachnoiditis which occurs secondary to intraventricular haemorrhage or meningitis.

Question 18
a. Coarctation of the aorta (CoA).
b. Absent femoral pulses but palpable brachial pulses.
c. Four limb blood pressure measurement.
   ECG.
   Echocardiogram.
   Cardiac catheterization.
d. Initially, prostaglandin infusion and/or a dopamine infusion.
   Definitive treatment is surgery.

COMMENTARY
a. The most likely diagnosis is CoA. This baby has many clinical features of congestive cardiac failure, namely sweating, tachycardia, gallop rhythm, tachypnoea, respiratory distress and hepatomegaly. You are told that the baby has brachial pulses but impalpable femoral pulses, which makes CoA more likely than hypoplastic left heart syndrome and other causes of congestive cardiac failure in the newborn. The X-ray features are compatible for CoA, but similar appearances are found in other conditions causing congestive cardiac failure.

b. Other investigations could include:
(i) Four limb blood pressure measurements. Classically in CoA the blood pressure in the arms is higher than in the legs.
(ii) ECG. This shows marked right ventricular hypertrophy.

(iii) Echocardiogram. The diagnosis of CoA can be confirmed on echo which can also look for additional cardiovascular abnormalities. Over half of all patients with CoA have an associated ventricular septal defect or aortic stenosis. In these cases one would expect a murmur to be audible.
(iv) Cardiac catheterization. This is required to show the extent and position of the CoA as well as the condition of the descending aorta.

c. A baby with a diagnosis of CoA should be treated with an infusion of prostaglandin. This may be life-saving and will maintain ductal patency allowing blood flow into the distal aorta. High doses of prostaglandin may cause apnoea requiring ventilation and most clinicians would therefore recommend elective ventilation if high dose prostaglandin is to be used. In severe CoA there is often renal compromise secondary to diminished renal blood flow. A dopamine infusion is therefore commonly used to improve renal blood flow. Definitive treatment of CoA requires surgery at a paediatric cardiac centre.

Question 19
a. Microcolon.
b. Hirschsprung's disease.
   Meconium ileus.
c. Rectal biopsy.
   Immunoreactive trypsin level in the blood.
d. Surgical excision for Hirschsprung's disease.
   Colostomy.

COMMENTARY
The contrast study shows a microcolon. These appearances suggest that this colon has not been used and is therefore narrow in diameter. The differential diagnosis is between Hirschsprung's disease and meconium ileus. The diagnosis of

Hirschsprung's disease is made histologically, showing an absence of ganglion cells in the nerve plexi. Rectal biopsy is therefore mandatory and can be partial thickness using the 'suction' technique or full thickness taken under general anaesthesia at the time of operation.

The treatment of Hirschsprung's disease is surgical with the formation of a colostomy and the removal of the aganglionic segment in the first instance. Colostomy reversal is carried out usually at around six months of age.

Up to 90% of infants with meconium ileus have cystic fibrosis. It is therefore important to test these infants for cystic fibrosis. This can be done in neonates by measuring the immunoreactive trypsin level in the blood if the child has not undergone gastrointestinal surgery or had a blood transfusion. Other methods include sweat tests and looking for genetic markers. Initial treatment of meconium ileus may be medical in the form of gastragraffin enemas; however most cases require surgical intervention with gastrograffin bowel washouts.

Question 20
a. Examine the baby's eye with an ophthalmoscope, directing the light at the pupil. You should be able to see a red reflex.
b. Cataract.
   Retinoblastoma.
c. Diabetes mellitus.
   Rubella infection.
   Cytomegalovirus infection.

COMMENTARY
a. Detection of a red reflex in a neonate is not difficult. You will require an ophthalmoscope and someone to hold the baby. If you are lucky the baby's eyes will be open. If so, all you need do is look through the ophthalmoscope lens directing the light at the baby's pupil and you will

see a red reflex. If the baby's eyes are closed, you should gently part the eye lid whilst looking through the ophthalmoscope. There is no place here for prising the eyelids open!

b. An absent red reflex is suggestive of a cataract or retinoblastoma. An absent red reflex is always an indication for an expert ophthalmological opinion.

Question 21
a. Tracheo-oesophageal fistula.
b. Cardiac disease.
   Anorectal anomalies.
   Intestinal atresia.
   Skeletal anomalies.
   Renal anomalies.
c. Pass a replogal tube and take a chest X-ray.
d. Surgery.

COMMENTARY
The baby should be kept nil by mouth and given intravenous fluids. Ideally a replogal tube should be placed in the upper pouch and aspirated continuously. If a replogal tube is not available a large nasogastric tube should be placed in the upper pouch and aspirated regularly instead. A chest X-ray should be taken with such a tube in position. This confirms the diagnosis of tracheo-oesophageal fistula and will also show evidence of aspiration. Some surgeons prefer contrast studies of the upper pouch to confirm the diagnosis but these are not essential. Blood samples for chromosome analysis should also be taken prior to surgery.

Question 22
a. Heart block.
b. May be associated with systemic lupus erythematosus.
c. Lupus anticoagulant.
   Anticardiolipin antibody.
   Anti-Ro antibody.
d. Recurrent miscarriages.

Intrauterine growth retardation.
Pre-eclampsia.
Unexplained intrauterine death.
Hypertension.
Abruptio placenta.

COMMENTARY
The ECG shows a ventricular rate of
50/minute with complete heart block.
Here the atria and ventricles are beating
independently of each other. The atrial
rate is therefore higher than the
ventricular rate confirming complete heart
block.

Congenital heart block may be due to
maternal connective tissue disease, in
particular systemic lupus erythematosus,
which may be subclinical. Although the
mother of this baby was not known to have
systemic lupus erythematosus she did have
a rash which may have been the rash
associated with lupus. All mothers of
babies with congenital heart block should
be screened for anti-Ro and anti-La
antibodies as a marker for a connective
tissue disorder.

Question 23
a. Septic screen
b. Anticonvulsants (IV phenobarbitone).
    Broad-spectrum antibiotics.
    Correct electrolyte imbalance.
c. Neonatal meningitis.
d. Group β-haemolytic *Streptococcus*.

COMMENTARY
a. This baby requires an urgent septic
screen including a lumbar puncture. As he
has clinical signs of sepsis and of cerebral
irritability with convulsions he should have
his electrolytes and blood sugar checked as
well as his serum calcium and magnesium.
Blood gas analysis should also be carried
out along with a cranial ultrasound scan
and an electroencephalogram.

b. Neonatal convulsions are a medical
emergency and require prompt

investigation and treatment:
(i) The convulsions should be treated with
an anticonvulsant, e.g. phenobarbitone
(20 mg/kg).
(ii) Once the septic screen is completed a
broad-spectrum antibiotic with good
cerebrospinal fluid penetration should be
commenced in order to treat any possible
meningitis.
(iii) Any electrolyte imbalance should be
corrected with intravenous electrolyte
replacement.

c. The most likely diagnosis is neonatal
meningitis, although clearly other causes of
convulsions need to be explored. The most
likely organisms are by late-onset group
β-haemolytic *Streptococcus* and Gram-
negative bacilli. Although there is a family
history of epilepsy in this case, idiopathic
epilepsy does not occur during the
newborn period.

Question 24
a. Bilateral talipes equinovarus.
b. Congenital dislocation of the hip.
    Meningomyelocele.
c. Simple exercise.
    Splinting in severe cases.
    Corrective surgery in very severe
      cases.

COMMENTARY
This infant has bilateral talipes
equinovarus with associated muscle
wasting of the lower limbs. Where this is
severe and bilateral the other anomalies
that should be actively sought include
congenital dislocation of the hip and
meningomyelocele. Mild positional talipes
equinovarus, where the foot can be
passively corrected to a neutral position,
requires simple exercises only. In the more
severe cases where the foot cannot be
passively corrected, splinting is needed
but the parents should be told that the
baby may ultimately require corrective
surgery.

Question 25

a. Clean the heel with an alcohol mediswab.

Hold the leg around the ankle with your thumb and fingers. Do not hold around the calf or this will cause bruising.

Prick the heel with a disposable lancet.

Collect the blood into capillary tubes or onto the Guthrie card.

Wipe away any excess blood.

b. The most medial and lateral portions of the plantar surface.

Part D
Revision Questions

QUESTIONS

Set one

1 Mrs PE is para 2+0 (both alive). One of her sons has cystic fibrosis. She is planning on having another child and has come to see you for some advice. Could you answer the following questions which she has for you.
a. What are the chances of her next child having cystic fibrosis?
b. Can this be diagnosed before the child is born? If so, when and how?
c. What are the complications of the test for such a diagnosis?

2 A young girl who has just had an ectopic pregnancy treated by salpingectomy has come to see you for follow-up.
a. What is the recurrence risk of the condition?
b. What contraceptive advice will you give her?
c. What further advice will you give her?

3 Miss JP has been on Femodene (containing ethinyl oestradiol and gestodene) without any problems for two years. She has recently read that this is one of the contraceptive pills that causes blood clots in women. She has come to see you with some questions.
a. What are the chances of developing a blood clot in her leg?
b. Are there any particular factors that increase the risk?
c. Are there any investigations that you can perform to ascertain the level of risk?
d. What are the warning signs of blood clots in one's legs?

4 A smear report from a 19-year-old patient has been reported as severe dyskaryosis.

a. What immediate advice will you offer her?
b. Name two methods of treating this condition locally. Give two complications of each method.
c. What is the long-term management of this patient?

5 A urine sample obtained from a patient at your antenatal clinic at 34 weeks' gestation showed nitrites and ++ proteinuria. Previous urinalysis at 26 weeks was reported as normal.
a. What two conditions may be responsible?
b. What further investigations will you perform on her (name three)?
c. What are the complications of these two conditions in pregnancy (give one for each of the conditions)?

6 Heather Brown has been to see you many times with lower abdominal pain in pregnancy and on each occasion, an MSU has grown *Escherichia coli* and *Pseudomonas* species.
a. How will you manage her from now onwards?
b. What additional investigations may you perform on her now and in the long term?
c. What is the likely cause of her recurrent urinary tract infections?

7 Figure 78 (see also colour plate section) was taken from a 37-year-old woman at surgery.
a. What is the diagnosis?
b. What symptoms may she have presented with (give three)?
c. What other treatment options could she have been offered (give two)?

8 A prenatal diagnosis was performed on a 30-year-old woman at 24 weeks'

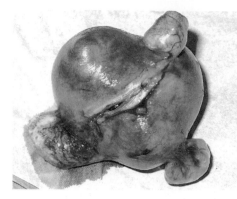

Fig. 78

gestation. The fetal karyotype was reported as 45XO.

a. What is the diagnosis?
b. What are the external features of this condition?
c. The woman wishes to know what the potential problems for the baby are (give two).
d. What might have been the indication for karyotyping?

9 Miss F is very anxious about her weight and facial hair which she finds very unsightly. She has come to see you for treatment.

a. Give two causes of this condition.
b. What two investigations will you perform on her?
c. What do you expect to be abnormal from these investigations?

10 Mrs D has been unable to conceive despite regular sexual intercourse for 2 years. She suffers from dysmenorrhoea and deep dyspareunia but her cycles are regular.

a. What are the differential diagnoses (give two)?
b. What investigation will you perform to help differentiate the two conditions?
c. What further investigations will you perform on her (give two)?

11 A 24-year-old para 1+0 was admitted at 38 weeks' gestation with constant lower abdominal pain and vaginal bleeding. Examination findings were: blood pressure 140/90, temperature 37.1°C, pulse 98/minute. The fundal height was 38 cm but the uterus was described as irritable.

a. What is the most likely diagnosis?
b. What investigations will you perform on this patient (give three)?
c. What will be the definitive management for her?
d. Name four complications of this condition.

12 Figure 79 shows a cream which has been given to your patient (on her very first visit) by a gynaecologist.

a. Give an indication for the use of this cream.
b. What symptoms may she have presented with (give three)?
c. What is a potential complication of this cream?
d. What are the contraindications for its use?

13 This is from a family planning clinic (Fig. 80).

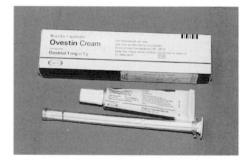
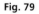

Fig. 79

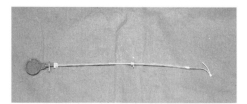

Fig. 80

a. Identify the method of contraception.
b. What is the failure rate?
c. What are the contraindications for this method of contraception (give three)?
d. What advice will you give the woman requesting it after counselling and insertion?

14 Mrs KD had a hysterectomy seven days ago. Her temperature is 38.5°C and her pulse is 90/minute.
a. What four symptoms may she have?
b. What four signs may she present with?
c. What four investigations may you perform?

15 A 34-year-old nulliparous woman has been to see you following the loss of her fourth pregnancy at nine weeks' gestation. The previous ones were confirmed pregnancies all between six and eight weeks. She is seeking your advice.
a. What is the most likely diagnosis?
b. What five investigations would you wish to arrange for her?
c. What are her chances of achieving a viable pregnancy (assuming all investigations are normal)?
d. What advice will you give her if the investigations are normal?
e. What would have been confirmatory of a previous pregnancy?

16 An ultrasound scan report on a 25-year-old primigravida at 35 weeks' gestation reads as follows: single fetus cephalic presentation, anterior placenta not low. BPD = 77 mm = 34.5 weeks, HC = 233 mm = 33.6 weeks. AC = 218 mm = 30.3 weeks, FL = 68 mm = 35 weeks. Liquor volume reduced – maximum pool depth is 1.5 cm. Fetal stomach, bladder and kidneys seen.
a. What is the diagnosis?
b. What two investigations may you perform on this patient?
c. How will you monitor this pregnancy from now onwards?

d. What three complications may arise from this condition?

17 Cynthia White has been told by the hospital that she has carcinoma of the cervix stage IIa.
a. What is carcinoma of the cervix stage IIa?
b. What three investigations does Cynthia require before treatment is considered?
c. If the condition is untreated, what four complications may arise?
d. What are the two treatment options for this patient?

18 Mrs D delivered a 3.7 kg male infant five days ago. She is becoming very weepy and the midwife has observed that her mood has changed.
a. What is the most likely diagnosis?
b. What three other symptoms may she have?
c. What treatment would you offer her?
d. What must you do before she is discharged from the hospital?

19 A 46-year-old nulliparous woman is keen to go on HRT.
a. What four questions must you ask her?
b. How may she take her HRT?
c. What three complications of HRT may she develop?

20 Mrs L complains of urinary incontinence. Her frequency and volume chart is shown in Fig. 81.
a. What is the most likely diagnosis?
b. What three further investigations will you like to perform on her?
c. What two treatment options may you offer her?

21 What two instructions would you give a patient in the following situations who wishes to start taking the combined pill?
a. A nulliparous woman.
b. Following a normal vaginal delivery.
c. Following a miscarriage or abortion.
d. Someone who has missed a pill.

Name:

Date	Time	Volume in (mls)	Volume out (mls)	Comments
18.5.97	0700	250 (coffee)	150*	Wet before going to the loo
	0800		20	
	0900	100 (coffee)	70	
	1000			
	1100		35*	Wet self
	1200		*	Wet self
	1300		75	
	1400	250		
	1500			
	1600		100*	
	1700		15*	Wet self
	1800		175	
	1900			
	2000		200	
	2100			
	2200			

Fig. 81

22 Fiona is a 25-year-old air hostess who is finding compliance difficult with the pill and is asking about Depo-Provera.
a. How does it differ from the combined pill?
b. What is the risk of pregnancy?
c. Is there any link with cancer?
d. What side-effects may occur?

Set two

1 This is an oral glucose tolerance test report from a 24-year-old primigravida at 28 weeks' gestation. Her blood glucose levels before pregnancy were normal.
Report: **Fasting = 5.5 mmol/l, 60 minutes = 10.4 mmol/l, 120 minutes = 9.2 mmol/l.**
a. What is the diagnosis?
b. Give three possible indications for this test in this patient.
c. What is the first line management for her?
d. Name four complications of this condition during pregnancy and labour.

2 A 35-year-old woman presented to your practice with painful, heavy and regular menstrual cycles of three years' duration.
a. Name three differential diagnoses.
b. What three investigations would you perform after a vaginal examination?
c. What medical treatment would you give her for the heavy periods? (Give two examples and the dosages.)

3 This microbiology report (Fig. 82) is from a woman at 16 weeks' gestation.
a. What treatment (dose and duration) will you offer her?
b. What advice will you offer her?
c. What are the side-effects of the drug you have prescribed?
d. What other investigation would you like to perform?

4 This is a cooperation chart (Fig. 83) from a woman who has just attended the midwife for antenatal care.
a. What is the most likely diagnosis?
b. What four important investigations would you perform on her?
c. What advice will you offer her in the community?

MICROBIOLOGY **pils**
REPORT

PUBLIC HEALTH LABORATORY
LEICESTER ROYAL INFIRMARY NHS TRUST
LEICESTER LE1 5WW
Telephone: 0116 254 1414 Ext. 6536/6546   Lab No.:

UNIT No.:
NAME:

SEX: DATE OF BIRTH:
SPECIMEN: HVS
SITE:
REQUEST:
BY:

DATE/TIME COLLECTED: DATE/TIME RECEIVED:

Culture(s)

No neisseria
No candida
Trichomonas vaginalis ++++
Few baceilli present

DATE/TIME TELEPHONED: DATE/TIME REPORTED: *Signature*..

Fig. 82

d. What further investigations may be performed in the hospital (give three)?

5 Identify each of these methods of contraception (Fig. 84) and for each one give two side-effects.

6 You have been called to see a woman at home who has not been able to void 24 hours after delivery.
a. What is your first line of management?
b. What investigation will you perform?
c. Name two causes of this condition.

7 Figure 85 shows a vital signs chart from a woman who delivered seven days ago.
a. What is your diagnosis?
b. Name four causes of the condition.
c. What two investigations will you perform on her?

8 This young woman is epileptic and is on Epilim 200 mg daily and wishes to become pregnant. She has come to see you for counselling.
a. What advice will you give her about her drug treatment during pregnancy?
b. What other advice will you give her concerning the management of her pregnancy?
c. What dietary advice will you give her?

9 A 26-year-old woman has been admitted with six weeks amenorrhoea, vaginal bleeding and a positive home pregnancy test. She has had two previous miscarriages at eight and seven weeks respectively. Vaginal examination showed an open os and a bulky uterus.
a. What immediate investigations will you perform?
b. What treatment will you offer?
c. Name four subsequent investigations that you will perform on her.

10 A 29-year-old woman at risk of HIV was referred at 16 weeks' gestation for counselling.

HOME VISIT BY MIDWIFE ☐ ☐ ☐ INITIALS								U·S SCAN
EARLY DISCHARGE/FULL STAY PREFERRED								
Treatment Remarks		Signature	Hb	Oes	H.P.L.			B.P.D. C.M.S.
Scan = Dates.								
well: good bn.								
well								
well et								
4o Swollen fingers Headaches								
SPECIAL POINTS (NB previous illnesses)		Blood Transfusion		V.D.R.L.				
		Sheffield No.		Rub.A/b				
		Blood Group		Rh.A/b				
		Rhesus		S.C.Screen				

PREFERRED HOSPITAL.....................

PREFERRED CONSULTANT ....

ANTENATAL RECORD

Date	Amen. (Wks.)	Fundus	Pres. Pos.	Relation pp to Brim	F.H.	Urine Gluc.	Urine Prot.	B.P.	Oed.	Weight kg.,	Return Visit G.P.	Return Visit Hosp.
28·4·9	12	—	·	—	—	—	NAD	110/60	—	82	4	
12·5·91	14					—	NAD	110/70	—	83		28 wks
25·5·91	16	16		—	—	—	NAD	115/75	—	84	4	
23·6·95	20	20		—	—	—	NAD	120/75	—	85	4	
20/7/95	24	24	—	—	fetal mov pat.	+	trace	120/70	—	86	8	
18/8/95	28	27cm	Ceph	free	LL	NAD	NAD	120/80	—	89	^	4/week
14/9/95	32	32	ceph	free	H	NAD	NAD	130/80	—	92	2	
28/9/95	34	33cm	ceph	4/5	LL	—	+	120/85	/	91	2	
13/10/95	36	34cm	Ceph	3/5	rt	—	++	140/95	+	95	2	

Menstrual History	6 / 28				Years married			Height		cm (NB >
Cycle	Date of last Cervical smear	3	10	94	FEEDING: BREAST		BOTTLE		UNCERTAIN	
Bleeding since LNMP	nil				CHEST X-RAY			RESULT		
Date hormone tablets ceased					DATE OF QUICKENING					

Fig. 83

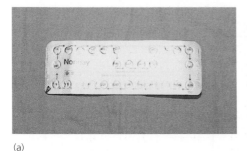

(a)

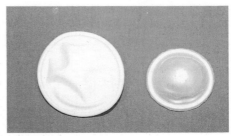

(b)

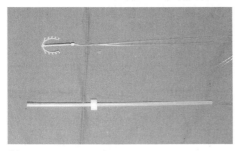

(c)

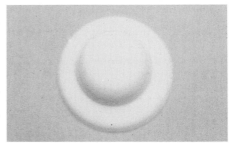

(d)

Fig. 84

a. Give four factors that increase the risk of HIV infection.
b. If she is HIV-positive, what is the risk of the virus being transmitted to the fetus?
c. Name two methods by which the virus can be transmitted to the baby.

11 A 17-year-old has come to see you for emergency contraception.
a. What two important questions will you ask her?
b. Name two methods of emergency contraception.
c. What advice will you give her for each of the methods?

12 A 26-year-old single G5P4 (all alive) who is still working presented with breathlessness at 36 weeks' gestation. There is nothing of significance in her past medical history. The midwife examined her and the fundal height was 32 cm. You do not feel that she has had a DVT/PE.

a. Give two possible causes of her breathlessness.
b. What investigation(s) will you like to perform (maximum of two)?
c. What will be your management plan/advice (immediate and long-term)?
d. When will you deliver the fetus?

13 A 38-year-old woman who has just had a total abdominal hysterectomy and bilateral salpingo-ophorectomy has come to see you with a letter from the hospital asking you to offer her HRT.
a. What three contraindications of HRT will you want to exclude?
b. What are the benefits of HRT (name four)?
c. What else will you do before putting her on HRT?
d. What are the complications of HRT (give two)?

14 You referred Mrs O to the hospital

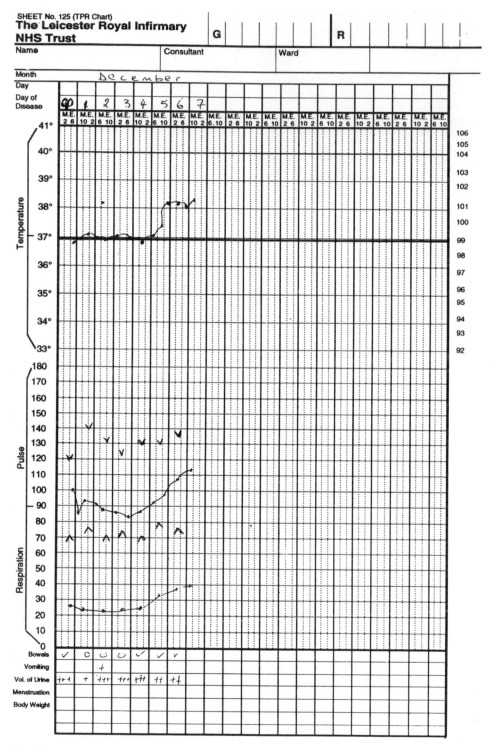

Fig. 85

because her fundal height was much bigger than her dates. She returned to you with this ultrasound picture (Fig. 86).

a. What is the diagnosis?
b. What are the complications of this condition in pregnancy (name four)?

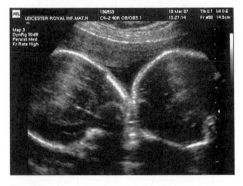

Fig. 86

Fig. 87

c. Name three other causes of a larger than dates fundal height.

15 A 24-year-old woman presented to your surgery with oligomenorrhoea and infertility. You requested a hormone assay. The results are shown in Fig. 87.

a. What three other symptoms may she have?
b. What is the diagnosis?
c. What other investigations will you perform?
d. What will be your first line of treatment?
e. How else might you achieve similar results?

16 Miss P is 18 years old. She has been to see you because of lower and right upper abdominal pain and a temperature of 37.5°C. She has had intermittent vaginal discharge for the past two months. An

W360	LEICESTERSHIRE PATHOLOGY SERVICE CHEMICAL PATHOLOGY		
Cons/GP & Location:	UNIT NUMBER:		SURNAME:
	DoB/Age:	Sex:	Forename:
	Patient Address:		

Specimen type: Lab No: Date & Time of report: 4.3.96

LH   = 14.0 iu/l
FSH   = 4.5 iu/l
Prolactin   = 265 miu/l
17 B estradiol = 237
Testosterone = 2.6
DHEAS   = 7.4

Comment:
Diagnosis: LMP = 3.3.96

T Bilirubin µmol/l 3-17	Alan. Trans. IU/l 2-53	Gamma G.T. IU/l 0-35f;50m	Alk. Phos. IU/l 40-130	Urate µmol/l 200,350f;500m	Phosphate mmol/l 0.8-1.4	T. protein g/l 60-80	Albumin g/l 35-55	Adj. Calci mmol/l 2.1-2.6
Sodium mmol/l 133-144	Potassium mmol/l 3.3-5.3	Bicarbonate mmol/l 22-30	Urea mmol/l 2.5-6.5	Creatinine µmol/l 60-120	Calcium mmol/l 2.1-2.6	Glucose mmol/l 4.0-6.6	Date & Time of Specim	
QUOTED REFERENCE RANGES ARE FOR ADULTS								

endocervical swab was positive for *Chlamydia* antigen.
a. What is the treatment for her?
b. What single important measure will you take?
c. What is the cause of her right upper abdominal pain?
d. What other investigations would you like to perform on her (name two)?

17 A 64-year-old obese diabetic presents with post-menopausal bleeding.
a. What three investigations may you perform on her?
b. Histology of the endometrial sample reveals grade 3 endometrial cancer. What is the treatment of choice?
c. What are the other two methods of treatment that may be considered?
d. What adjuvant therapy may she be offered if indicated?

18 A 28-year-old woman is booked for antenatal care in your practice. Her alpha-fetoprotein is reported as 3 multiples of the median (Mom), i.e. raised.
a. What are the causes of such a report? (Name four.)
b. What further investigation will you perform on her?
c. What are the possible complications of this pregnancy assuming that all investigations are negative (give two)?

19 A 22-year-old woman who had a coil fitted two years ago, attends for a routine cervical smear. During the procedure you notice that the coil threads are not visible.
a. What questions would you like to ask the patient?
b. What action would you take?
c. What immediate advice would you give the patient?

20 Sharon is a 15-year-old attending her GPs surgery requesting hormonal contraception. She had unprotected sexual intercourse with a new boyfriend 60 hours ago and is very worried about pregnancy. She refuses to involve her parents and is concerned about confidentiality.
a. What are the legal considerations?
b. Discuss the treatment regimen.
c. What are the important side-effects of the treatment?
d. What is the known failure rate?
e. Is there any risk to the fetus in a continuing pregnancy?
f. What follow-up would you advise?
g. What other advice would you give?

Set three

1 Ms JJ is a 19-year-old secretary who booked for antenatal care at 11 weeks and whose booking ultrasound scan showed a cyst measuring 11 × 16 cm arising from the left ovary. The cyst had internal reflective echoes and some solid areas. The right ovary was normal.
a. What is the likely diagnosis?
b. What will be your plan of management?
c. What are the potential complications of this cyst in pregnancy?
d. What is the main risk of operating early?
e. What is the main risk of surgery?

2 A 65-year-old gravida 0 presented to the gynaecology clinic with abdominal discomfort, dyspeptic symptoms and an abdominal mass. On examination, she was found to be cachectic but not pale. There was a relatively immobile non-tender mass arising from the pelvis. There was associated ascites.
a. What is the likely diagnosis?
b. What further investigations would you like to carry out?
c. Assuming your diagnosis is confirmed, what will be the treatment of choice?
d. What are the risk factors for this condition in this patient?

3 A 26-year-old G3P1 presented with abdominal pain, mild vaginal bleeding, reduced fetal movements and dizzy spells at 38 weeks' gestation. On examination: she was pale and sweaty, pulse 110/minute, blood pressure 95/50.
a. What is the most likely diagnosis?
b. What other clinical signs may she have?
c. What investigations might you perform?
d. What fetal complications may arise from this complication?
e. What three maternal complications may arise from this condition?

4 Figure 88 (see also colour plate section) was obtained after termination of a pregnancy at 30 weeks' gestation.
a. What is the most likely diagnosis?
b. How might the diagnosis have been made?
c. What factors may indicate the need to scan for this complication?
d. What are the risk factors for the occurrence of this condition?
e. How may the occurrence of this condition be reduced?

5 A 26-year-old housewife who has been married for six years is complaining of lower abdominal pain during menstruation. She has given you the following gynaecological history:
LMP: 18 May 1997
Menstrual cycle: 3–5/28–30, regular, heavy with clots on days 2 and 3

Menarche: 13 years
Parity: 0 + 0
Contraception: nil
Pain: duration three years
Relationship to period: start two days before menstruation and lasts for up to three days after cessation of period
Associated deep dyspareunia.
a. Give two differential diagnoses for this patient.
b. What other symptoms may she have presented with?
c. What three investigations will you perform?
d. What two treatments will you offer for each of your differential diagnoses?

6 Miss Clark presented with six weeks amenorrhoea, abdominal pain and vaginal bleeding. On examination, she was clinically stable but tender in the left vaginal fornix. An ultrasound scan of the pelvis showed an empty uterus and a thickened endometrium. Both ovaries were visualized.
a. What other four investigations may she require?
b. What are your two differential diagnoses?
c. What treatment options may you offer her?

7 Figure 89 shows a type of contraception.
a. What is the name of this method of contraception?

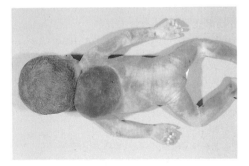

Fig. 88

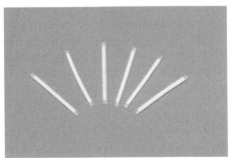

Fig. 89

b. To which group of contraceptives does it belong?

c. How is it administered?

d. List four known complications of this method of contraception?

e. Give three contraindications for its use.

8 Figure 90 shows a product.

a. What is this product used for?

b. Name two contraindications to its use.

c. What are the benefits of this treatment (give four)?

d. In which group of patients is it most suitable?

e. How else may a similar therapy be administered?

9 Mrs B is a 57-year-old woman referred to the gynaecology outpatient clinic with irregular vaginal bleeding. She was found to have a bulky uterus on vaginal examination. An ultrasound scan showed a 12 mm thick irregular endometrium. A biopsy was obtained and the histology report was as follows: 'well-differentiated adenocarcinoma of the endometrium'.

a. What is the treatment of choice?

b. Give five risk factors for endometrial carcinoma.

c. In general, what factors determine prognosis?

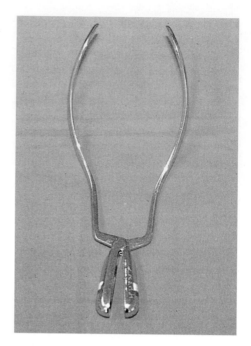

Fig. 91

d. What adjuvant therapy may she be offered?

10 Figure 91 shows an instrument.

a. What is the name of this instrument?

b. Give two indications for its use.

c. What five conditions must be fulfilled before its application?

d. List two complications that may result from the use of this instrument.

11 This report (Fig. 92) was obtained from a 35-year-old Afro-Caribbean primigravida with a bossing skull and a history of bone pain crises at 34 weeks' gestation in her first pregnancy.

a. What is the most likely diagnosis?

b. What three features in the report support your diagnosis

c. What two further investigations would you like to perform on her?

d. What treatment might you offer her?

e. Name three complications that may arise from this condition in pregnancy.

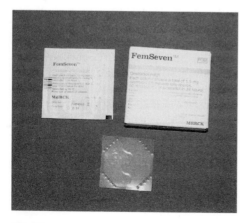

Fig. 90

LEICESTERSHIRE HAEMATOLOGY SERVICE			Tel. ext: LRI 6530: LGH 4566: GGH 3575							

Consultant + Patient Loc. or GP Name + address			SURNAME				FORENAME			
			SEX F	DOB/AGE 31/10/68			HOSPITAL No.		LABORATORY No.	

Differential	Neutrophils	Lymphocytes	Monocytes	Eosinophils	Basophils	Atypical Lymph.	Metamyelo	Myelocytes	Pro. Mye	Blasts
WBC % x 10⁹/1	76.0	16.9	4.9	1.8	0.4					
	6.84	1.52	0.44	0.16	0.04					
% Adults Normal Range ABS	40-75 2.0-7.5	20-45 1.5-4.0	2-10 0.2-0.8	1-6 0.04-0.4	1 or less 0.01-0.1					

Machine Differential	Granulocytes	Lymphocytes	Mononuclears	WHITE CELL COMMENT						
WBC %										
	%	%	%							

EXCLUDE Fe DEFICIENCY

QUOTED NORMAL RANGES ARE FOR ADULTS

Hb	RBC	HCT	MCV	MCH	Reticulocytes	WBC	Platelets	P.V.	Date of Sample 12/11/96
M 13.5-18.0 F/1.5-16.5	M 4.5-6.5 F 3.9-5.6	M 0.4-0.54 F 0.37-0.47	80-99	27-32	0-2	4-11	150-400	1.5-1.72	Date Reported 12/11/96
*8.9	4.12	*0.282	*68.4	*21.6		9.8	202		Run 87 Page 1 of 1
g/dl	x 10¹²/1		fl	pg	%	x 10⁹/1	x 10⁹/1	cp	

Fig. 92

12 Figure 93 shows a cooperation card from a primigravida at 34 weeks' gestation.
a. What is the most likely diagnosis?
b. Name four investigations that you might like to perform on this patient.
c. Give three complications of this condition.
d. How may you monitor the patient?

13 This is an investigation (Fig. 94) which has been ordered on a multigravida at 36 weeks' gestation and was commenced on 12/3/97.
a. What is the investigation called?
b. What does it show?
c. What advice will you offer the patient?
d. What are the possible complications of this pregnancy?

e. How else may this pregnancy be monitored?

14 A grand multipara delivered seven days ago and has presented with vaginal bleeding.
a. What is a grand multipara?
b. What may be the cause of the bleeding?
c. What signs might you elicit on pelvic examination?
d. How may she be investigated?

15 A mother who delivered three days ago has developed pleuritic chest pain associated with difficulties with breathing.
a. What is the most likely diagnosis?
b. What blood investigations will you perform on her
c. What other investigations would you like to perfom?
d. How may she be treated?

HOME VISIT BY MIDWIFE ☐☐☐ INITIALS					U·S SCAN
EARLY DISCHARGE/FULL STAY PREFERRED					

Treatment Remarks	Signature	Hb	Oes	H.P.L.	B.P.D. C.M.S.
F M F					
Good Fm.					
Fm ✓					
well, good FM.					

SPECIAL POINTS (NB previous illnesses)	Blood Transfusion	V.D.R.L.
	Sheffield No.	Rub.A/b
	Blood Group	Rh.A/b
	Rhesus	S.C.Screen

PREFERRED HOSPITAL ....

PREFERRED CONSULTANT ....

ANTENATAL RECORD

Date	Amen. (Wks.)	Fundus	Pres. Pos.	Relation pp to Brim	F.H.	Urine Gluc.	Urine Prot.	B.P.	Oed.	Weight kg.,	Return Visit. G.P.	Return Visit. Hosp.
25·11·96	8 +					N A0		110/60		63kg	10	
9·12·96	11 +			Seem =	Dols		NA0	120/55		64kg		36
28·1·97	18	18			FHA Easicn	+	NA0	110/70		65kg		
11·2·97	24	24		FHH with Sonicaid	+		Nil	105/65		66kg		
24·4·97	28	28	Ceph	free	AH3	NA0		120/70	+	69kg		
19·5·97	34	33cm	Ceph	free	AHHL		NA0	150/45	++	75kg		

Menstrual History			
Cycle 5/28 Date of last Cervical smear	12	95	
Bleeding since LNMP none			
Date hormone tablets ceased			

Years married 4	Height 165 cm (NB ›
FEEDING: BREAST	BOTTLE	UNCERTAIN
CHEST X-RAY	RESULT
DATE OF QUICKENING	

Fig. 93

Hospital: "KICK CHART"

Date Kick Chart commenced: Name:

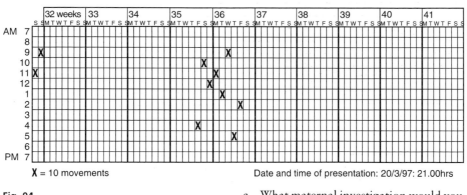

X = 10 movements   Date and time of presentation: 20/3/97: 21.00hrs

Fig. 94

e. What four pre-pregnancy risk factors may she have had?

16 This is a CTG (Fig. 95) obtained from a primigravida who presented in labour at 38 weeks' gestation.

a. What does the CTG show?

b. What further investigations would you like to perform on the fetus?

Fig. 95

c. What maternal investigation would you like to perform?

d. Give one fetal cause of this type of CTG?

e. What may be the causes of this fetal condition?

f. What other causes may be responsible for this type of CTG?

g. What is the prognosis in this fetus?

17 Figure 96 (see also colour plate section) shows a specimen obtained at surgery from a 26-year-old asymptomatic woman

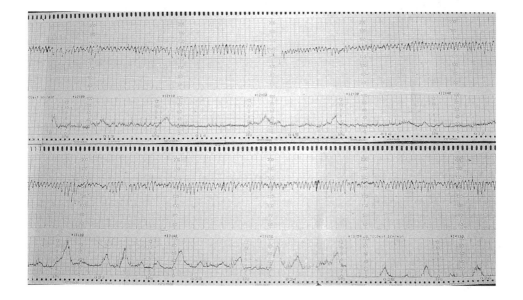

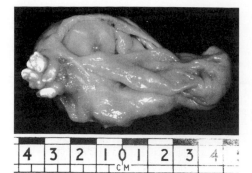

Fig. 96

referred by her GP because of an incidental pelvic mass felt during the insertion of an intrauterine contraceptive device.
a. What is the most likely diagnosis?
b. What two investigations might have diagnosed this pathology?
c. What other symptoms may she have had?
d. What is the treatment of this condition in pregnancy?

18 Figure 97 (see also colour plate section) was taken from a 42-year-old woman.

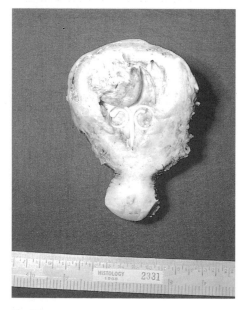

Fig. 97

a. What does the photograph show?
b. When was the specimen obtained?
c. What symptoms may the patient have presented with?
d. What other method of treatment could she have been offered?

19 Figure 98 (see also colour plate section) was taken after a termination of pregnancy at 12 weeks' gestation.
a. What does it show?
b. Give three common causes of this abnormal pathology.
c. What important investigation should have been performed on the fetus?
d. What might have been the reason for scanning the patient early apart from booking?

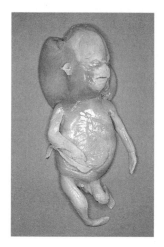

Fig. 98

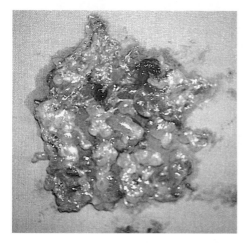

Fig. 99

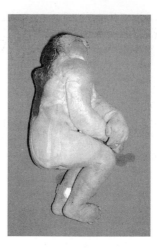

Fig. 100

20 A 31-year-old woman in her second pregnancy presented at eight weeks' gestation with irregular vaginal bleeding. The uterus was 10 weeks in size and the cervical os was opened. An evacuation for an inevitable miscarriage produced this specimen (Fig. 99, see also colour plate section).

a. What is the most likely diagnosis?
b. What symptoms might have led to the suspicion of this diagnosis?
c. What two investigations might be useful in this condition and what abnormalities would you expect?
d. Give two pathological types of this condition.

21 A 19-year-old primigravida had a termination of pregnancy at 28 weeks' gestation and the fetus is shown in Fig. 100 (see also colour plate section).

a. What abnormalites can you identify?
b. How might the diagnosis have been made?
c. Give two markers of this condition.
d. How may its recurrence in subsequent pregnancies be reduced?

ANSWERS

Set one

Question 1
a. One in four.
b. Yes, by chorionic villus sampling at 10–13 weeks' gestation or amniocentesis after 11 weeks.
c. Miscarriage.
    Ruptured membranes.
    Rhesus isoimmunization if rhesus-negative.
    Infection.

Question 2
a. Ten times greater than in a woman who has not had an ectopic pregnancy.
b. Avoid using an intrauterine contraceptive device or progestogen-only contraceptive.
    May use a barrier method of contraception.
    May use a combined oral contraceptive pill.
c. Report early if her period is missed.

Question 3
a. Unless there are risk factors, the risk is about 3 : 100 000.
b. Obesity.
    Family history.
    Previous deep venous thrombosis.
    Smoking.
    Thrombophilia.
c. Protein C and S levels.
    Antithrombin II levels.
    Factor V Leiden.
d. Pain in the calf.
    Swelling of the calf.

Question 4
a. Refer for colposcopy.
b. LLETZ: haemorrhage, stenosis and infection.

Laser: haemorrhage, stenosis and infection.
Diathermy: infection and stenosis.
Cold knife cone biopsy: haemorrhage, infection, stenosis, dysmenorrhoea infertility and cervical incompetence.
c. Follow-up for at least five years with smears.

Question 5
a. Urinary tract infection.
    Pre-eclampsia.
b. MSU, MCS.
    Full blood count.
    Urea and electrolytes/uric acid.
    Liver function test.
    Blood pressure.
c. *Pre-eclampsia*:
    Preterm labour.
    Eclampsia.
    Intrauterine growth retardation.
    Abruptio placenta.
    HELLP syndrome.
    UTI:
    Preterm labour.
    Chronic pyelonephritis leading to scarring and hypertension.

Question 6
a. Place her on prophylactic antibiotics.
b. Arrange a renal ultrasound scan.
    Arrange an intravenous pyelogram 3–4 months after delivery.
c. Congenital malformation of the kidneys.
    Renal calculi.

Question 7
a. Multiple uterine fibroids.
b. Menorrhagia.
    Abdominal mass.
    Pressure symptoms.
    Dysmenorrhoea.

c. Myomectomy.
   LHRH analogues.

Question 8
a. Turner's syndrome.
b. Short stature.
   Webbed neck.
   Widely spaced nipples.
   Wide carrying angle of the upper
      limbs.
c. Infertility.
   Amenorrhoea (primary).
   Coarctation of the aorta.
   Short-statured.
d. Cystic hygroma.
   Family history of chromosomal
      abnormalities.
   Maternal age.
   High Down's risk.

Question 9
a. Polycystic ovarian disease.
   Adrenal hyperplasia (tumour).
   Cushing' syndrome.
b. Follicle-stimulating hormone (FSH).
   Luteinizing hormone (LH).
   Testosterone.
   Ultrasound scan of the ovaries.
   Adrenocorticotrophic hormone.
c. Testosterone high.
   Altered LH : FSH ratio.
   Peripheral cysts in the ovary.

Question 10
a. Endometriosis.
   Pelvic inflammatory disease.
b. Diagnostic laparoscopy.
c. HVS.
   Endocervical swab.
   Luteal phase progesterone. Tubal
      patency tests (HSG, laparoscopy and
      dye test or HyCoSy).

Question 11
a. Abruptio placenta.
b. Full blood count.
   Coagulation screen.
   Urea and electrolytes.

Group and save.
CTG.
c. Deliver the baby.
d. Disseminated intravascular
      coagulation.
   Fetal distress.
   Intrauterine death.
   Postpartum haemorrhage.
   Renal failure.

Question 12
a. Atrophic vaginitis.
   Atrophic cervicitis.
   Prolapse before surgery.
   When changing pessaries.
   Urinary incontinence.
b. Dry vagina.
   Post-menopausal bleeding.
   Post-coital bleeding.
   Superficial dyspareunia.
c. Endometrial carcinoma.
   Irregular vaginal bleeding.
d. Cancer of the endometrium.
   Breast cancer.
   Recent deep venous thrombosis or
      pulmonary embolism.
   Undiagnosed vaginal bleeding.

Question 13
a. Copper-7 intrauterine contraceptive
      device.
b. 3–4 per hundred women years.
c. Previous ectopic pregnancy.
   Pelvic inflammatory disease.
   Allergy to copper.
   Unexplained uterine bleeding.
   Pregnancy.
d. To check string after each period.

Question 14
a. Generalized abdominal pain.
   Chest pain.
   Cough.
   Wound discharge.
   Pain in the calf.
   Dysuria.
   Frequency of micturition.
b. Crepitations.

Calf tenderness.
Swollen calf.
Red and tender wound.
Discharge from wound.
c. MSU.
Chest X-ray.
Swabs.
Ultrasound scan of the calf.
Venogram.

Question 15
a. Recurrent miscarriage.
b. Parental chromosome analysis.
Hysterosalpingography.
Infection screening (viral, protozoal
    and bacterial).
Early follicular phase FSH and LH.
Anticardiolipin antibodies.
Lupus anticoagulant.
c. Up to 70%.
d. Try for a further pregnancy.
e. Ultrasound evidence of pregnancy.
Histological evidence of chorionic villi
    in products of conception.

Question 16
a. Asymmetrical intrauterine growth
    retardation.
b. Doppler velocimetry of umbilical and
    middle cerebral arteries.
CTG.
Biophysical profile.
c. Serial ultrasounds for growth checks.
Serial CTGs.
Serial Doppler scans.
Serial biophysical profiles (BPP).
Fetal kick chart.
d. Intrauterine death.
Fetal distress.
Preterm delivery.
Necrotizing enterocolitis.
Polycythaemia.
Neurodevelopmental disability.
Long-term morbidity from
    hypertension, heart-attacks and
    diabetes mellitus as adults.

Question 17
a. Cancer in the cervix and upper two-

thirds of the vagina, but the pelvic side
wall is free.
b. Staging.
Ultrasound scan of the kidneys.
CT scan.
Urea and electrolytes.
Full blood count.
Group and crossmatch.
Liver function test.
c. Renal failure.
Haemorrhage.
Infection.
Vesico-vaginal fistula (VVF).
Recto-vaginal fistula (RVF).
Distant metastasis.
Death.
d. Radical surgery.
Radiotherapy.

Question 18
a. Puerperal blues.
b. Insomnia.
Poor appetite.
Irritable.
Palpitations.
c. Reassurance.
Sedation.
Supportive care.
d. Notify GP/Community midwife.

Question 19
a. Past history of breast cancer.
Previous deep venous thrombosis.
Hysterectomy.
Liver disease.
Previous pulmonary embolism.
b. Orally.
Implants.
Gel.
Transdermal patches.
c. Deep venous thrombosis.
Breast tenderness.
Breast cancer.
Endometrial cancer.
Endometrial hyperplasia.
Weight gain.

Question 20
a. Detrusor instability.

b. MSU.
   Blood glucose.
   Cystoscopy.
   Cystometry.
   Examination for prolapse.
c. Anticholinergics.
   Physiotherapy.
   Bladder retraining.
   Oestrogens.
   Calcium channel blockers.

Question 21

a. Start on/before the 4th day of cycle.
   If starting later, use additional
   precautions during the first 14 days.
b. If breast feeding avoid combined oral
   contraceptives.
   If not breast feeding, can start within
   first week though commonly women
   are asked to wait for 2 weeks.
c. Start immediately or within first 3 days.
   If starting later, use additional
   precautions for 2 weeks.
d. Take it as soon as remembered and the
   next one at the normal time.
   If more than 12 hours (especially with
   the first in the packet), continue but
   take extra precautions for 7 days. If 7
   days run into the next pack, do not
   have the pill-free interval and start
   the next pack immediately.

Question 22

a. A progestogen-only contraceptive
   may be used when there is a
   contraindication to oestrogens.
   It is given by IM injection every 12
   weeks.
   It is more suitable when there are
   compliance problems.
b. Ranges from zero to one per hundred
   women years.
c. Protects against endometrial cancer.
   No increased risk of cancer of the
   cervix, liver or ovaries.
   Inconclusive evidence about a slight
   increase in the incidence of breast
   cancer.
d. Cycle disruption – initially one-third of

women have frequent prolonged
bleeding; with continued treatment
55% become amenorrhoeic at
12 months and 68% by 24 months.
Delay in return of fertility – on average
eight months after the last injection.
There is no permanent infertility with
83% of women conceiving by 12
months.
Weight gain due to increased appetite
(average 0.5–2 kg in the first year).
Androgenic effects may occur, e.g.
acne.
Occasional backache or depression.

Set two

Question 1

a. Impaired glucose tolerance.
b. Obesity.
   Family history of diabetes mellitus.
   Persistent glycosuria.
   Polyhydramnios.
   Recurrent vulval boils.
   Recurrent vaginal candidiasis.
c. Dietary control.
d. Polyhydramnios.
   Unexplained fetal death.
   Fetal macrosomia.
   Obstructed labour (shoulder
   dystocia).
   Increased risk of caesarean delivery.

Question 2

a. Uterine fibroids.
   Endometriosis.
   Pelvic inflammatory disease.
   Dysfunctional uterine bleeding.
b. Ultrasound scan of the pelvic
   organs.
   Diagnostic laparoscopy.
   Full blood count.
   High vaginal and endocervical swabs.
c. Tranexamic acid 0.5–1 g four times a
   day.
   Combined oral contraceptive pill.
   Danazol 200 mg twice a day.
   Synarel 200 µg twice a day.

Question 3

a. Metronidazole 400 mg three time a day for seven days.
b. Avoid alcohol.
   Avoid sexual intercourse.
c. Headaches.
   Nausea and vomiting.
d. *Chlamydia* test.
   Screen for *Neisseria gonorrhoeae*.

Question 4

a. Pre-eclampsia.
b. Full blood count.
   Urea and electrolytes.
   Urinalysis.
   Liver function test.
c. She needs hospital assessment/admission.
d. Twenty-four hour urine protein.
   Ultrasound scan for growth and liquor volume.
   Doppler velocimetry of the umbilical artery.
   Biophysical profilometry.
   Cardiotocography.

Question 5

a. Noriday.
   Side-effects: menstrual irregularities; nausea; vomiting; headaches; breast discomfort; depression; weight changes.
b. Diaphragm.
   Side-effects: allergy/hypersensitivity to rubber in device; increased liability to urinary tract infections.
c. Multiload copper intrauterine contraceptive device.
   Side-effects: perforation of the uterus; expulsion; pelvic infections; menstrual abnormalities; ectopic pregnancy; lower abdominal pain.
d. Cervical cap.
   Side-effects: hypersensitivity to device.

Question 6

a. Catheterize and examine the perineum.
b. MSU.
c. Bladder atony secondary to labour.

Perineal haematoma.
Trauma secondary to instrumental delivery.
Fistula formation after obstructed or instrumental delivery.

Question 7

a. Puerperal pyrexia.
b. Breast infection.
   Urinary tract infection.
   Abdominal wound infection.
   Chest infection.
   Deep venous thrombosis.
c. Full blood count.
   MSU.
   Chest X-ray.
   Venogram.
   Doppler of the vessels in the calf.
   Electrocardiogram (ECG).

Question 8

a. May change treatment to another less teratogenic antiepileptic.
   May need to increase dosage during pregnancy.
   Increased risk of neural tube defects.
   Must continue with medication as the risk of fetal problems is greater without treatment than with treatment.
b. Anomaly scan will be offered at 18–20 weeks' gestation.
c. Need to take folic acid before pregnancy and up to 13 weeks' gestation.

Question 9

a. Full blood count.
   Group and save.
b. Evacuation of the uterus.
c. Lupus anticoagulant.
   Thyroid function test.
   Anticardiolipin antibodies.
   Maternal and paternal karyotype.
   Hysteroscopy/hysterosalpingogram/ HyCoSy.

Question 10

a. Intravenous drug abuses.

Bisexual partner.

Partner from Africa/Asia in the last 12 months.

Haemophiliac.

b. 25–30 per cent transmission.

c. During childbirth.

During breast feeding.

Question 11

a. Date of last menstrual period.

When did she last have sexual intercourse?

b. PC4.

Intrauterine contraceptive device.

c. PC4: take two tablets and another two after 12 hours. If there is any vomiting, repeat the tablets. If a period is missed, report to the doctor.

Intrauterine contraceptive device: this will be inserted within five days of sexual exposure.

Question 12

a. Exhaustion.

Anaemia.

b. Full blood count.

Scan for fetal growth and liquor volume.

c. Advise her to give up working.

Refer to the hospital.

Kick chart.

Serial growth scans/Doppler/CTGs.

d. When any serial monitory investigation indicates, but certainly before 40 weeks (if scans confirm severe intrauterine growth retardation).

Question 13

a. Active pulmonary embolism.

Active oestrogen-dependent malignancy (breast cancer, endometrial cancer).

Active liver disorders.

Undiagnosed breast lump.

b. Prevents osteoporosis.

Prevents cardiovascular diseases.

Prevents atrophic vaginitis.

Reduces psychosomatic problems of menopause.

c. Examine her breasts.

d. Endometrial hyperplasia.

Deep venous thrombosis.

Breast tenderness.

Breast cancer.

Question 14

a. Twin pregnancy.

b. Antepartum haemorrhage.

Anaemia.

Preterm labour.

Polyhydramnios.

Premature rupture of fetal membranes.

Pressure symptoms.

Intrauterine growth retardation.

c. Polyhydramnios.

Wrong dates.

Pelvic tumour.

Large fetus.

Question 15

a. Obesity.

Hirsutism.

Acne.

Male-type baldness.

b. Polycystic ovarian disease.

c. Ultrasound scan.

Semen analysis.

Tubal patency test.

d. Induce ovulation with clomiphene citrate or gonadotrophins.

e. Laser of the ovaries.

Diathermy of the ovaries.

Wedge resection of the ovaries.

Question 16

a. Doxycycline.

Ciproxin.

Azithromycin.

b. Contact tracing.

c. Perihepatic infection with *Chlamydia trachomatis* (Fitz–Hugh–Curtis syndrome).

d. Endocervical, urethral and rectal swabs for other sexually transmitted diseases.

Question 17

a. Ultrasound scan of the pelvic organs.

Endometrial biopsy.
Hysteroscopy.
b. Total abdominal hysterectomy and bilateral salpingo-ophorectomy.
c. Radiotherapy.
Therapy with progestogens.
d. Progestogens.

Question 18
a. Threatened abortion.
Intrauterine death.
Twin pregnancy.
Neural tube defects.
Cystic adenomatous malformation of the lungs.
Congenital nephrosis.
Anterior abdominal wall defects.
Sacrococcygeal teratomas.
Idiopathic.
b. Fetal detailed ultrasound scan.
c. Intrauterine death (unexplained).
Intrauterine growth retardation.

Question 19
a. Has she noticed coil expulsion?
Was her last menstrual period normal and what was the date?
How long have the threads been absent (assuming she self-examined)?
Has she noticed any unusual symptoms?
b. Probe the cervical canal gently with Spencer Wells forceps to search for the threads.
If the threads are not found in the cervical canal, sound the uterine cavity (if in follicular phase only).
Arrange for an ultrasound scan.
c. Use alternate contraceptive until the scan result is available.
Return to see you with scan result.

Question 20
a. Gillick competence.
Advise her to discuss with her parents.
Respect her rights to confidential treatment.
b. Two tablets of ethinyl oestradiol 50 µg

and levonorgestrel 250 µg (PC4) now.
Repeat 12 hours later.
c. Nausea.
Vomiting.
d. One to five per cent.
e. There is no evidence of any fetal risk.
f. Return if there is amenorrhoea after three weeks.
g. On-going contraception.
Safer sex.

Set three

Question 1
a. Dermoid cyst.
b. Arrange for the cyst to be removed at 14–16 weeks' gestation.
c. Tortion.
Rupture.
Obstructed labour.
Malpresentation.
d. Miscarriage from removal of the corpus luteum of pregnancy.
e. Uterine contractions followed by miscarriage.

Question 2
a. Ovarian carcinoma.
b. Abdominal ultrasound scan.
Intravenous urogram.
Full blood count.
Urea and electrolytes.
CA125.
CT scan.
c. Total abdominal hysterectomy, bilateral salpingo-ophorectomy, omentectomy (debulking surgery) and adjuvant chemotherapy.
d. Age.
Parity.

Question 3
a. Placental abruption.
b. Fundal height greater than dates.
Tender uterus.
Fetal parts difficult to palpate.

Absent fetal heart beat.
c. Full blood count.
Coagulation screen.
Group and crossmatch.
Urea and electrolytes.
Cardiotocography.
d. Fetal distress.
Intrauterine death.
Fetal anaemia.
e. Disseminated intravascular
coagulation.
Renal failure.
Maternal death.
Courvelier uterus with severe
postpartum haemorrhage.

Question 4
a. Spina bifida.
b. Ultrasound scan.
c. Raised alpha-fetoprotein.
Hydramnios.
Previous affected baby.
d. Previous affected baby.
Epileptic on sodium valproate.
e. Maternal intake of folic acid
pre-conception and up to 12 weeks'
gestation.

Question 5
a. Endometriosis.
Pelvic inflammatory disease.
b. Infertility.
Vaginal discharge.
c. Haemoglobin estimation.
High vaginal and endocervical swabs.
Diagnostic laparoscopy.
d. Endometriosis: hormone treatment and
surgery.
Pelvic inflammatory disease: antibiotics
and surgery.

Question 6
a. Full blood count.
Group and save.
β-HCG.
Diagnostic laparoscopy.
b. Ectopic pregnancy.
Follicular cyst.

c. Salpingectomy.
Salpingostomy.
Treatment with methotrexate.
Injection with hypertonic solutions or
prostaglandins.
Conservative management if there are
follicular cysts.

Question 7
a. Norplant.
b. Progestogen-only contraceptives.
c. Subdermal implant.
d. Irregular vaginal
bleeding/amenorrhoea.
Acne.
Hair loss.
Weight gain.
Headaches.
Loss of libido.
e. Unexplained vaginal bleeding.
Pregnancy.
Active liver disease.

Question 8
a. HRT.
b. Active oestrogen-dependent cancers.
Active deep venous thrombosis or
pulmonary embolism.
Active liver disease.
c. Protection against osteoporosis.
Cardioprotective.
Prevention of vasomotor symptoms.
Prevention of atrophic urogenital
changes.
Protection against early onset of
Alzheimer's disease.
d. Post-menopausal women.
e. Orally.
Implants.
Vaginal rings (E-string).
Gels.

Question 9
a. Total abdominal hysterectomy and
bilateral salpingo-ophorectomy.
b. Nulliparity.
Obesity.
Diabetes mellitus.

Polycystic ovarian disease.
Oestrogen-producing ovarian tumours.
Hypertension.
Early menarche and late menopause.
c. Degree of differentiation.
Extent of myometrial invasion.
d. Therapy with progestogens.
Radiotherapy.

Question 10
a. Wrigley's forceps.
b. Delay in second stage due to maternal
exhaustion.
Fetal distress in second stage.
Maternal cardiorespiratory problems
necessitating assisted delivery.
To deliver the head at caesarean
section.
c. Cervix must be fully dilated.
Membranes must be ruptured.
Uterus must be contracting.
There must be no contraindications to
vaginal delivery.
Presentation must be suitable.
Analgesia must be adequate.
Operator must be skilled.
Bladder must be emptied.
d. Trauma to the genital tract.
Trauma to the bladder.
Trauma to the fetus.

Question 11
a. Iron-deficiency anaemia and sickle-cell
anaemia.
b. Low haemoglobin.
Low mean corpuscular volume.
Low mean corpuscular haemoglobin
concentration.
c. Serum ferritin.
Haemoglobin electrophoresis.
Stool for occult blood and hook worms.
d. Iron and folic acid and, if there is no
response, blood transfusion.
e. Intrauterine growth retardation.
Pseudotoxaemia of pregnancy.
Bone pain crises.
Acute sequestration crises.
Recurrent urinary tract infections.

Question 12
a. Pregnancy-induced hypertension/pre-
eclampsia.
b. Full blood count.
Liver function test.
Urea and electrolytes and urates.
Urinalysis.
MSU.
Ultrasound scan.
c. Eclampsia.
Intrauterine growth retardation.
Preterm delivery.
Intrauterine fetal death.
Disseminated intravascular
coagulation.
Renal failure.
Liver failure.
Cerebrovascular accident.
d. Four-hourly blood pressure checks.
Serial full blood count, liver function
test, urea and electrolytes and urates.
Twenty-four-hour urinary protein.
Serial fetal growth scans.
Serial fetal monitoring (CTGs,
Dopplers).

Question 13
a. Fetal kick chart.
b. Less than 10 fetal movements within a
12-hour period on the ninth day.
c. To report to the hospital for fetal
assessment.
d. Intrauterine fetal death.
Fetal distress in labour.
e. Doppler velocimetry.
Biophysical profile.
Daily CTGs.

Question 14
a. Someone who has had at least five
pregnancies progressing beyond 24
weeks' gestation.
b. Retained products of conception.
Endometritis.
c. Foul-smelling vaginal discharge/lochia.
Open cervical os.
Tender uterus/adnexa.
d. Full blood count.

Group and save serum.

Ultrasound scan.

HVS.

Question 15

a. Pulmonary embolism.

b. Blood gases.

c. Chest X-ray.

ECG.

Venogram.

V-Q scan.

d. Intravenous heparinization initially.

Warfarin for at least six weeks after the initial heparinization.

Streptokinase.

e. Thrombophilia.

Family history of deep venous thrombosis/pulmonary embolism.

Previous deep venous thrombosis/pulmonary embolism.

Obesity.

Question 16

a. A sinusoidal pattern.

b. Fetal blood sampling for fetal haemoglobin, pH and acid–base status.

c. Kleihauer Betke test.

d. Fetal anaemia.

e. Severe rhesus disease.

Fetomaternal haemorrhage.

Ruptured vasa praevia.

f. Thumb sucking (but this should not be as long lasting as this).

Severe fetal hypoxaemia.

g. Perinatal mortality is 50–75%.

Significant morbidity (severe neurodevelopmental disability).

Question 17

a. Dermoid ovarian cyst.

b. Ultrasound scan.

Plain abdominopelvic X-ray.

c. Intermittent lower abdominal pain.

Dull ache.

Acute abdominal pain.

Features of thyrotoxicosis.

d. Surgical removal.

Question 18

a. An intrauterine contraceptive device in the uterus.

Submucous fibroids.

b. At hysterectomy.

c. Heavy periods.

Vaginal discharge.

Intermenstrual periods.

d. Removal of the device.

Resection of the fibroid polyp.

Question 19

a. Large cystic hygroma.

b. Turner's syndrome.

Trisomy 21.

Trisomy 18.

c. Karyotyping as 75% of such fetuses have abnormal karyotypes.

d. Previous chromosomally abnormal fetus.

Family history of chromosome abnormality.

Patient's request.

Question 20

a. Hydatidiform mole (molar pregnancy).

b. Exaggerated symptoms of pregnancy (hyperemesis gravidarum).

Symptoms of thyrotoxicosis.

Passage of vesicles per vaginam.

c. β-HCG levels very high.

Ultrasound scan showing an enlarged uterus with a snow-storm appearance and no definite fetus.

d. Partial hydatidiform mole.

Complete hydatidiform mole.

Question 21

a. Spina bifida.

Anencephaly.

b. Ultrasound scan.

c. Raised maternal serum alpha-fetoprotein.

Polyhydramnios.

d. Maternal intake of folic acid pre-pregnancy and up to the end of the first trimester.